Journey Home

Samuel McLeod

Copyright © Samuel McLeod, 2015

All rights reserved. No part of this publication may be reproduced, stored in a retrieval system, or transmitted in any form or by any means—electronic, mechanical, photocopying, recording or otherwise—except for brief passages for the purposes of reviewing, as stated by the Canadian copyright law and the U.S. copyright law, without prior permission of the author.

ISBN: 978-0-9950941-0-9

ABOUT THE AUTHOR

Samuel McLeod is a witty storyteller born in a small village in eastern Canada. His exploratory nature has taken him on a life of adventure while pursuing Truth and leading him to an inexplicable Inner Peace. Sammy's participation in the material world as a businessman caused him to look beyond it, with a strong desire to gain an understanding of it.

Sammy's study of the mystical, the spiritual and the material has spanned over fifty years and brought him into many experiences in different countries throughout the world.

He is a certified teacher of Bija Meditation, an acknowledged Gran Master in Reiki Jin Kei Do, accomplished in many healing energies, including our planetary Archangels. Sammy's careers have been diverse from farming to mining, carpenter work and his love of real estate as a certified Business Broker & Commercial Realtor.

During the past 10 years of his life, Sammy has spent time in Africa, Colombia, Ecuador, Peru & Bolivia with Spiritual Masters, Shamans, Healers & Apus from different Tribes and Cultures. Each moment spent was one step closer, until an understanding and purification brought liberation to his heart so that he could once again experience life flowing freely from Spirit Energy.

GRATITUDE

I give thanks to Mother Earth (Mahii/Gaia) for this moment that we all share experiencing the beauty of our planet (Urantia). May she continue to guide us each day to become more human, kinder, more generous, more accepting, and more loving to each other. I live in gratitude for that spark of life within me that is beyond name, that mystery Who gives adventure to our beingness, the Source of all life. To that wonderful presence that is Love, Light, Beauty and Goodness, I take a breath and bow my head in reverence to Him, through His grace He gives us our first and last breath.

An earthly journey seldom concludes without a long list of souls who have assisted along the Way, mine is no different. I thank my brothers and sister who were always there for me and my parents who let my spirit run free, never imposing too many limitations on my decisions. I thank my son and my daughter for limitless support and love. The Warrior and the Fairy Queen have had to watch me stumble along somedays, yet never bailed out on me, what more could one ask of his children. I thank my stepson for always trying to understand me without judgment and for his quiet nature. They are all ancient souls, deep waters in their own way, they are friends, and it is wonderful to be able to share this experience with them.

One has many teachers along the Way but there are two that have demonstrated character through action, always giving and never asking anything in return. Maestro Zuluan Orion was here to help me wake up and give me sufficient tools to continue the journey on my own and for that and much more, I thank you Zuluan.

Joey is one of those rare beings, who never wavers in his friendship. He always has a sympathetic ear, ready to listen but never to repeat the words received in confidence. He genuinely enjoys the success and happiness of others and gives them a heartfelt congratulations when the opportunity arises. It has been an honor and a pleasure to call him my friend. Anymore that I say will only fall short, thank you Joey.

I thank Creator and the work of our guides, for bringing Rishi into my life, to complete each other so that we may journey together once again as companions. She is my teacher, my guide, my friend, life partner and my guru. She is my Orator of worlds beyond, a storyteller of dreamtime that gives meaning and understanding to this moment that we are experiencing. To be within her sphere of love is more than enough…

PREFACE

What is our purpose here on planet Earth? Have we come of our own accord? Perhaps that is part of our Soul's journey or adventure to find the answers to these questions and many more. More importantly though is our opportunity to become aware of who we are through the discovery and integration with your Thought Adjuster. Our Creator's desire to experience life throughout the Universes gives rise to each soul's individuality. It is here in our three-dimensional time space on Mother Earth where life seems to hurdle its challenges at us causing us to look for some meaning to it all.

Life can lose its pizazz along the way, only we know the intensity of it, no other can see life from our perspective, so we really journey alone. Creator brings us all home through an understanding of our Unity and Oneness, so any feeling of loneliness dissolves into something beautiful, beyond perception.

The game is set, earth is the stage where we play our parts ready or not, consciously, or unconsciously. The controllers of the game seem to have the upper hand as their energy grids, programming and cultural differences keep us asleep and predictable, reaping in their material gain. They demonstrate their force (causing fear) to take away our power, we have the free will to give it away or take it back, so there is no blame. We are responsible to wake up.

If you are searching for some answers, then you are most likely looking to get out of the game or at least step out of it long enough to know what it is, so that you can once again begin to play your part consciously. It will take some effort to remove the programming in this body we are born into as well as the mental, physical, and emotional memories accumulated over one's lifetime, but there in this unfoldment awaits your power.

If it is your time and intention to be free once again, then continue on, in knowing that all that is required will be shown to you each step of the way and as you reconnect to our fountain of life there you will encounter liberation, your graceful Heart, your Source.

TABLE OF CONTENTS

Early Days on the Farm 1
Memories of School 13
A Time for Change 25
Fork in the Road 31
Dream On 41
Countryside to the City 51
Restaurant – Tough School 61
Creator's Hand 75
Network Marketing Returns 85
A Real Fork in the Road 101
Final Years in Canada 107
The Call to Ecuador 117
Mahabharata 131
Life in Cuenca 137
Maestro Sat Guru 145
Maestro in Ecuador 159
Love Changes All 181
Jungle Life 201
Southern Cross 227
The Final Ceremony 261

EARLY DAYS ON THE FARM

It was in the mid-nineties on the hood of a white Ford Explorer, somewhere in Kentucky that this Traveler had come to the end of the road trying to face life on his own. He had had big dreams since a young age, but at thirty-eight years old he was completely worn out with no clear vision in sight. It was not a last resort decision, but it seemed liked the most promising and besides that, it felt right. God's presence was not new to this man but handing his life over to HIM sparked some anxiety in his heart.

Let us go back a bit to the mid-fifties of the twentieth century, to the birthplace of this story, a moment in time space for Traveler. This place is a small village called Martintown nestled in the eastern counties, home to many descendants of French, English, Dutch and Scottish immigrants. Many families arrived in Canada hundreds of years before and many more after the end of the 2nd World War. Life was simple, no cell phones, no computers, no Internet, just neighbor helping neighbor and for the most part, everyone was content.

Samuel McLeod

Martintown has over two hundred years of history, many people from this village and surrounding area settled here to begin a new life, a fresh start, perhaps difficult at times but at least free of the control and hardships that they were leaving behind. The main road that runs through the center of the village was once an Indian trail, situated above the flood plains of the river. The Indigenous not so long ago, freely roamed the area between the mighty St. Lawrence River to the South and the Ottawa River to the North. Change in life is inevitable; but rarely does it affect each person equally and as is the case many times, one gaining freedom while taking it from another. At least the Registry Office still has the area titled under Indian Lands, but they have long since disappeared or been moved to government granted Reserves.

There is still much of the Aboriginal existence in this area waiting to be discovered, on many farms the stone fences hold an abundance of treasures such as stone arrow heads, hatchets and stones used for tanning animal hides. According to the Treaty, this land was traded in exchange for some of the Islands on the St. Lawrence which became the Indigenous Reserve. Traveler's father spent one summer upon his return from duty in WWII, surveying these Islands with the Band's Indigenous Chiefs. Perhaps the land titles are in place, but there is still some bitterness harbored in a few Aboriginal families, over the loss of land, loss of life and their loss of freedom. Many Indigenous children were removed from their homes on the Reserves, up until the eighties and nineties, so that they could be educated in English, often without consent from their family or simply put into foster care.

As the early settlers became established, Martintown became a vibrant commercial center. The river runs through the heart of the Village and was once used to power the Grist Mill which remains a landmark. Local farmers would bring in their grain throughout the year to be ground into flour for baking or into feed for their livestock. There was a Sawmill on the banks of the river on the north end of town along with a casket maker and three General Stores supplying goods to the area. The original covered wooden bridge used during the horse & buggy days has since been replaced. Sitting on the steel bridge was a favorite summer pastime of Traveler along with a few friends, watching what little traffic there was, but at least they got to wave at their neighbors. Although the village only had a population of three hundred or so, it was home to three churches in the early days, Presbyterian, Protestant and Catholic.

The Aboriginal trail gave way to the dirt streets lined with plank sidewalks and hitching posts along the main street from east to west. Today the main road travels over a new bridge which was built along with a Dam, complete with a fish ladder to accommodate the Spring spawn of species coming up from the St. Lawrence. The main road going east to the Province of Quebec or west towards Toronto exhibits some of the most beautiful farms in eastern Ontario. There definitely seems to be something that feels so peaceful when one sees a herd of fifty or sixty Holsteins or Herefords, grazing in knee high grass in an open field, well perhaps not if you have to milk the dairy cows twice a day.

At the age of six months in 1956, Traveler moved to a fifty-seven-acre farm of rolling hills, stoned filled hills that would become his family home until 1985. This home is a two-story red brick house located just west of the village. It sits on a hill that is one of the highest points between the St. Lawrence River and the Ottawa River. Traveler is the youngest of his family of three brothers and one sister. The move was the beginning of fulfilling their parent's dream to become full-time farmers. Through the memories shared around the kitchen table the oldest brother Hugh laughs at the humiliation he experienced driving the Farmall tractor through the village with all the family's worldly possessions in tow on the farm wagon. To be allowed to drive the tractor at twelve years old was motivation enough for Hugh, even though he had to slide from side to side on the steel seat to be able to alternate between the clutch and brake, just in case he had to stop.

Life experiences here on Mother Earth seem to be by design, unfolding each lifetime in perfection. Traveler was not awake to this idea yet; this would come later, much later.

Traveler's first recollection of life was at the age of three playing with a toy tractor on the neighbor's farm. Many early memories were over at their place taking turns riding their pony Trigger in a pasture north of the dairy barn. They even learned how to jump into the saddle from behind, just like Roy Rogers. Robin and Don had forts that were constructed in the hay mow, a great place for hiding and becoming aware of an excitement they called fear. Life was shared with animals, an abundance of nature, family and neighbors who depended on each other in good times and in bad. Growing up caring for animals seem to help Traveler with the acceptance of life and death as being a natural part of existence. Unknowingly for Traveler, it was the beginning of detachment and covering up any emotion about death or pain.

The sixties seem to be a time of change and expansion on the farm as oil fired space heaters in the homestead were replaced with a new centrally located furnace and by the mid-sixties a new red & white International tractor was sitting in the driveway waiting to be admired by neighbors and family.

Local carpenters Kenny and Cecil began the construction of a new loafing barn on the home farm complete with a horizontal silo for feed storage and a feeding station that could accommodate sixty or seventy head of feeder cattle. They were like Laurel and Hardy as Kenny's tall frame stood straight as an arrow with suspenders holding up his denim coveralls and Cecil who was smaller in stature but ever present with his wit.

Lunch time was a moment for laughter as Kenny and Cecil would share their pranks such as Kenny leaving a fish to rest on the motor of Cecil's car while it seemed at the same time Cecil was throwing one in the trunk of Kenny's car and neither one catching on until the inevitable odor began to seep out. The expression on their faces described every detail of the event and then they lived in anticipation of their next prank. A story that remained with them was the time when Kenny bit into Penny's fresh apple pie, now Penny was well known for her delicious pies, and they were the highlight of any meal. Penny seemed to retain her youthful look and nature throughout her life. She could prepare a meal in no time and serve it while remaining tuned to the conversation round the table. Back to Kenny, Kenny couldn't wait for the first bite of pie and slide the loaded fork into his mouth but being absorbed in conversation he had not noticed Penny taking the pie directly from the oven, with her slightly burnt oven mitts, to the table. Kenny began to mumble as he rolled the hot pie from one side of his mouth to the other hoping to cool it down, this performance had all of them in tears and of course Kenny was too polite to unload the pie, even his tanned face turned red.

Traveler often would see his father on his knees praying before the Sun came up and he now wonders if the prayers were for prosperous times or strictly prayer in hope that the family car would make it home safely from the weekend trip to Quebec. The province of Quebec was only a short drive and drinking Ale in the local pubs there seemed to be open to anyone who at least looked sixteen or had enough money to buy a beer. Traveler's brothers were now driving, and father Sam had fresh memories of the tow truck bringing home yet another family car to rest on the stone fence, west of the house. Penny was no stranger to prayer either surely with a concerted effort of faith and gratitude their family survived its years of youth.

Traveler was very aware of God from a young age through the teachings of his parents and the example that they set in the community, they all lived the illusion of God being separate from them, that is what the priests were delivering in their Sunday sermons. Most families were devoted to God through prayer and attending Mass on Sunday. Everyone in Traveler's family always wore their best clothes on Sunday and Marlene would have her hair done up in Ringlets ready for what seemed to be a Sunday morning ritual. Traveler wasn't sure whether Marlene was trying to practice meditation during mass on Sundays or not but almost always she would faint during the Sermon, and usually Father Sam would be quick enough to catch her before she tumbled into the back of the next pew, but not always. In a community where faithfuls of the United Church, Presbyterian and Catholic religions practiced their beliefs, it seemed certain that they all believed in the same God, but a God who was separate from them. Even though at that time while seemingly praying to a God in the Heavens, Traveler felt a special relationship with Him.

Childhood on the farm brings nothing but wonderful memories for Traveler, maybe apart from his mother explaining to him that Santa Claus did not exist. He could not believe that just a few months before that heart-breaking news Santa had come bearing gifts, twice on Christmas Eve. Looking back, he could see the illusion, brother Hugh had returned home from British Columbia with more disposable money than the family had experienced before which allowed for a bountiful amount of Christmas gifts. Hugh always had a business sense which perhaps derived from a perceived necessity to maintain his impeccable appearance. He would on occasion hold a sell-off in his bedroom of unwanted clothing, the eager clients were Jimmy and Roddy along with their sister Marlene, if she had an interest. The intent was to upgrade his wardrobe with newer fashions. Hugh remains in fashion today although the sell-off is buried in time. Back to Christmas Eve, the tradition was that Traveler would go to bed for a while before going to mid-night Mass, then into bed after returning from church, and off to the land of dreams with thoughts of Santa's arrival in the night.

This year was different, when little Traveler came downstairs from his Christmas eve nap and ready for Mass, there were so many beautifully wrapped gifts under the tree, and everyone agreed that Santa had indeed already made his visit. First thing, the next morning when he slid down the banister Traveler was in for another surprise, this Christmas tree was now bearing at least double the number of gifts than the night before. He was convinced that Santa had for sure been to their house twice and how lucky he was. The next trip to Grandfather's farm was an opportunity to share the story with his Uncle John who laughed and agreed that it was good fortune and that he must have been a good boy.

Christmas was by far the most special time of the year in their family and their community as every family prepared for weeks to make this celebration of the birth of Jesus a special one. In their schools, their churches and in their homes, they were constantly reminded of the true purpose of this celebration.

This love and peace that was felt during that time each year could not be duplicated. Only we know the special relationship that we have with God and His Creator son, there is no doubt that this personal union exists. From a young age Traveler felt this uniqueness of being, but perhaps he was not aware of the presence of God within, that was causing this feeling.

As life on the farm evolved memories of past experiences remained vivid. One of Traveler's most favorite times was climbing the majestic Maple tree which stood alone on a hill centered on the highest point of their farm. This Maple with her strong arm like branches reaching up to the sky in reverence to a higher source seemed to have an unexplainable presence. He would sit up high on one of the branches, well cradled in place with his eyes closed enjoying the breeze and the warmth of the Sun whether it was Spring, Summer or Fall the experience was always blissful. Life, as it unknowingly happens to many, would slowly cloud over this connection that Traveler enjoyed in his youthful innocence.

They were given responsibilities at a young age which for Traveler included bagging grain with his sister Marlene on Saturday mornings. They were always hurrying to finish the job so they could go back into the house to catch the last hour or so of Bugs Bunny or another favorite cartoon. Most Saturdays they were given extra chores which delayed this enjoyment but one Saturday each month father Sam had to attend a meeting which allowed them to finish up early and return to the warmth of their family home.

During the Winter months the cattle were kept in the loafing barn so there were extra chores required to feed, bed them & ensure a fresh supply of water. After the cattle had been given their hay and grain Traveler would sit in the hay mow breathing in the crisp Winter air with his eyes closed, listening to the harmony of all the cattle chewing their meal with contentment. This moment seems simple now, but the feeling was unmistakable that of nothingness, just the rhythmic sound bringing a peaceful state.

Their awareness seemed to be heightened as to the importance of chores when they trekked to the barn during a Winter storm to be greeted by snow covered faces waiting for their breakfast. This daily work seemed all the more rewarding when they shared the conditions of the day with the cattle, feeling a part of their existence and sensing the fragility of life, one dependent on the other.

Raising cattle had its' blissful and rewarding moments but there were also trying times. In the Summertime fixing fences and chasing cattle seemed to be a weekly routine. There was always a leader in the group who managed to find the weak link in the fence and squeeze through onto greener pastures or more often to dine in the neighbor's corn field. At the end of the harvest, they would settle for any damages with a wagon load of corn or a discount in the invoice for combining.

Summertime was a season for gathering and preparation for the upcoming Winter. Looking back, they seemed to be taking in hay for most of the Summer depending on the amount of rain and the quantity of the crop. Stooking hay was probably Traveler's least favorite job right after the dreaded task of picking stones. Father Sam had lost most of hearing capability as a child after being dragged by his horse through the field and perhaps the remainder after marriage although around the kitchen table he missed nothing. Traveler rode the stooker on the rolling hills of Blackadder's farm and father Sam drove the International hydro-shift tractor with the baler & stooker in tow. He would normally have the first three bales neatly piled waiting for the next bale to come out the chute, only to turn around and see them sliding off onto the ground. Many times, he was not quick enough to reload the bales while trying to catch up with the baler so he would yell at his father to stop but to no avail. The initial thought was to throw a stone at him, but better judgment prevailed so instead he developed a shrill sounding whistle which seemed to snap Father Sam out of his seat and make them both laugh, a good break from the sweat of the day. At lunch time Penny would test out her newly acquired driving skills and bring a meal to the field allowing them to regenerate & get ready for the next round. There is nothing like a picnic to bring harmony back into your life and on the farm much needed patience.

Speaking of patience brings brother Rod to mind along with a couple of stories. Unfortunately, the farming community has far too many accidents with machinery and livestock causing injury or sometimes death. Rod was riding on the back of the tractor one morning, while standing on the drawbar with Father Sam at the wheel, Rod slipped and started sliding up the rear tire underneath the fender. You can imagine of course Rod screaming at his father to stop but you remember, Father Sam's hearing. Rod had two fears racing through his head, one of death and the other, was getting in trouble from his father for falling off the back of the tractor but fortunately Father Sam had wonderful peripheral vision and saw him out of the corner of his eye enabling him to stop the tractor in time.

Many years later Rod was home from university, his time away had neither cooled his temper, nor developed his patience, maybe that class was not offered. Rod, like Kenny in this story, carried his almost 6` frame quite well, quiet lean and a little mean, holding much of his Ancestor's warrior memory. Today was the day; it was time to move the cattle down the road from the home farm to the east place where they would spend the Winter. Rod was already mentally preparing for mishaps during the move which would inevitably delay his evening out with his friends. All was going well as the cattle raced along at a good pace down the Kings Road, the last hurdle was to steer the cattle into the corral, if they missed that turn then they were heading for the river which was a half a mile away. Traveler might have been the weak link in this cattle drive, trying to guide fifty or so steers. Whatever the reason, the cattle saw their chance at freedom and yes, a run to the river. Anticipating Rod's fury and perhaps from heightened nerves Traveler began to laugh as Rod chased him into the front field where the pigs were pastured. At thirteen he thought that he could fly, probably because he was light enough to make it possible. He could run fast and jump fences, but it was inevitable that he was doomed. Rod caught him in the middle of the field but to feed his frustration Traveler kept laughing, the rest of the story was not all that pretty but Rod did manage to stop Traveler's laughter, after fifteen grueling minutes or so, which included a short flight from above Rod's extended arms.

This event is only remembered from stories around the kitchen table at their home. Hugh who had a date lined up that evening with his girlfriend was called to rescue the prize boar from the manure pit which held about 4 feet of liquid slurry and as luck would have it the pit was full to the brim. Hugh had the task of trying to slip a rope around the pig's body so they could lift it out to safety with the front-end-loader. This animal was probably well over five hundred lbs., so the rope was its' only chance for survival. The boar was pulled to safety but left one lingering problem. The smell of hog manure is quite friendly but once it festers in the lagoon for a while it becomes almost impossible to remove the odor and only time can assist the process. Hugh had been dipping his hands in the lagoon trying to get the rope around the boar and now he was upstairs in the bathroom at their family home furiously scrubbing his hands. He would smell his hands after each fresh round of soap & rinse and the only comment was "Jesus" as Hugh dropped them back into the sink for one last try.

Life was rather good up until now, not too many bruises and lots of laughs…

MEMORIES OF SCHOOL

Traveler was never sure if he was born shy or when the dreaded challenge entered his life, but it became his biggest hurdle. His Mother had him ready for school, new clothes, lunch box loaded and out the door in knowing that he was the last child at home to begin this process. Their farm was about one mile from the Public School in Martintown and during the first couple of years Traveler rode with Mrs. Christie his 1st grade teacher. He can still see her green Studebaker Roadster coming down the road and certain that he could still recognize the scent of her perfume if it existed today. His Mother's enthusiasm about little Traveler's first day at School ended around Noon as he walked in the kitchen door to inform her that he had quit school. He knew that they were not allowed to walk on the road, so it was a trek through the neighbor's fields.

Traveler actually came to like school and looked forward to finishing homework and seeing the results of his efforts. Playing pranks and having fun seemed to be a part of his being right from the beginning of school. Not thinking about the consequences, he caught a couple of flies during class one day and set them on Mrs. Christie's chair, yes, his ride to school, and of course as the class waited with anticipation, she sat on them and spent most of the morning adorning her new accessories. Fear set in when she finally located the flies, after much giggling throughout the class had alerted her. Oh, that feeling of fear, how it can change one's experience. Without warning the question that drained the life out of Traveler was, "who did it?" before he could clear his mind Easter and Gail blurted out, we all did which seemed to bring the rest of the class in unison, coming to his rescue. To his relief Mrs. Christie decided to carry on with the class rather than investigate any further. That was close…

Father Sam was a trustee on the School Board which meant a visit to all schools in the district and each classroom at least once a year. Traveler always felt pride as his father walked into the class. He had lost most of his jet-black hair shortly after university, but his stature was that of a boxer who had developed his mass while working in the mines to help pay for his tuition. He had won his golden gloves in New York and his talent as a fighter remained with him well into his sixties. His sharp mind was an asset not only to be used in the science of boxing but in developing the area schools. The teachers would have some of their student's best work displayed and reminded them of the respect they needed to show the Board members. The teachers had a good relationship with the trustees, and all had the interest of education as being most important. There did not seem to be any of the teachers during this time that ever fell short on fulfilling their role as examples and mentors to the students.

Discipline in the classroom for the students was twofold, one being respect for the teachers and the other being respect for their parents. The teachers had a certain leeway to ensure that students stayed the course and didn't disrupt the classroom during their studies which occasionally meant a rap on the knuckles from the wooden pointer, although many times they were quick enough to slide their hand to safety. The school's principal, Helen, usually managed to wrap them in the end, she was relentless. Each student seemed to know the limits, but a few liked to live on the edge, as Bob Proctor has often repeated, if you're not living on the edge, you're taking up too much room.

Each morning before class began, they repeated the Lords' prayer and then sang "God Save the Queen" as Canada did not have its own national anthem yet. It seemed to be a good way to get the student's minds centered and ready to start the day.

Looking back most families including Traveler's, had truly little money but most were oblivious to the fact because it was just normal for most everyone. Their interests were playing games or sports and looking for the next adventure after school. In the Spring of the year when the water was high it was home to test out the log raft, left behind by his brothers. All was fine unless he happened to fall into the pond and then it was home to change which usually meant being greeted by Penny to receive that dreaded drink of ginger in punishment for playing where he had been told not to.

Spring was a time when the Pickerel and Suckers would swim up the local river from the St. Lawrence reaching the Martintown Dam to spawn. There was so many you could lay down on the rocks and catch them with your hands. As is often the case, it was not long before the Conservation Officers were putting a stop to this enjoyment, a little more control.

Most Winters, depending on the amount of snow, brought a time where they were able to skate on the ponds or on the river. Freezing temperatures never seemed to be an issue as they dressed for the day and enjoyed the crisp Winter air. Jack Frost usually started creating his magic in December with trees and fences covered with a heavy frost which would glisten as the morning Sun began to rise. Many mornings Jack managed to do both panes of glass on the windows of the farmhouse, yep, fresh mornings stepping out of the sack. In their youth they wanted to get out and enjoy each moment with all the beauty it brought but then as the years slipped by, most preferred to watch from the window and the warmth of their home, same view perhaps but a much different experience.

Youth usually remains free of any thoughts of worry about tomorrow or of any lack in their life. Children enjoy all of creation each new day without any preconception of how it will unfold. As they began to express or experience more from the memories of the body that they are born into, perception changes. The programming engrained by their parent's, done unconsciously, along with that of society, done intentionally, begin to anchor them more and more into the physical world, perceiving it to be all that is. While their mind/body begins to take control of their experience, the nature of their true existence is less and less prevalent. It is through ignorance or misunderstanding that this illusion begins in our life and normally through disillusion of the same or some painful moments that the journey begins from darkness to light, looking for what is Truth or real.

It was time at last to make the transition from childhood to that of a teenager and step into the new world of High School. Traveler's sister Marlene had one year left to finish before going off to university so at least he had someone for guidance just in case the experience was too overwhelming. He stepped off the bus at school and was greeted by the sound of motorcycles which were being parked at the north end of the parking lot. There were a couple of brand spanking new 650 Triumphs, an older BSA and a couple of 750 Nortons, all sparkling for their first impression of the school year. He along with most of his friends were tipping the scale at about one hundred and thirty-five lbs. and the lads climbing off their bikes were an easy six-foot wearing cowboy boots and towering over them like they were misplaced from kindergarten. Fortunately, they had been through their own experience of starting High School and were not too hard on the boys, allowing them some time to adapt to their new surroundings.

Traveler enjoyed High School immensely with many good friends and he always maintained the thought in his mind, that finishing Grade twelve would be his ticket to freedom, ready to make his mark in this world. They would have the odd session with Chucky their Guidance Teacher to share thoughts on a career path, maybe an Airline Pilot or join the Army. Some days he felt that the teaching staff were expecting him to follow Marlene or Rod who were attending University, but it just was not registering. Jimmy had just returned from a four-year tour with the Army, home for a few months and then off to live in the United States. Traveler barely knew Hugh who was in British Columbia striking out on his own. Ah what the heck, there was too much fun to be had no time to think about the future, not just yet.

I mentioned that Traveler was not sure where or when his shyness began or took hold of him, but it was evident that it was well rooted in his teenage years. One experience which may have kicked started a few issues was during his first communion in the Catholic Church. There were a couple of facts at that time that he was unaware of, one was that his family were Catholic, but he attended the Public School and to make the situation worse his father was a Trustee on the Board. He never would have guessed that the Nuns who taught at the Catholic School across the street could take their bitterness about those facts out on him. It was the worse feeling of rejection that he had felt up until that time and it planted the seed of self-doubt deep into his being.

It is unfortunate that religion, which is supposed to be the very source of guidance to a relationship with God or Creator, could also be a source of rejection. Perhaps the Nuns had not quite grasped the teachings about judgment yet, oh well, neither had Traveler.

Being shy is, in his mind, one of the worst emotional restrictions to have to carry with you in life, only himself or someone else that lives with it can understand its' perceived power. The thought of having to stand in front of the class to give a short speech or tell a story would overpower the enjoyment of any other thought and create a feeling of fear, almost paralyzing. It was bad enough that he felt nervous about walking back to his seat from communion, during Sunday mass, let alone having to speak in front of his classmates. This energy or nervousness seem to bring out humor in his speech as his mind raced trying to take the focus away from the task at hand. This performance kept classmates occupied in laughter, but this was a temporary fix, as the feelings of fear and self-doubt continued to grow. It did not help the teachers much either, as they liked to maintain some essence of order in the classroom.

Having grown up in an area where drinking was the norm, Traveler was no stranger to alcohol and the effects of this mind-altering refreshment. He had watched his family and their friends enjoy this tradition of drinking at every gathering, any cause for celebration, and as time went on, he had experienced it firsthand. His first glass of scotch was probably at the age of ten or eleven while watching his parents playing Bridge with the Samson's. Father Sam liked his Scotch neat with a two-finger measure in the glass, yes, the pinky & the index. Traveler began sipping on the Scotch as the card game progressed and within a short period of time, he had licked it all up. Penny was soon guiding him up the stairs to bed, but he began to feel the effect just before hitting the last few steps, quickly tucked into the sense of another world, spinning him into deep sleep. It was the first glass of scotch but not his last.

The first craving came at the Family reunion held on his Grandfather's Farm where Uncle John & his family lived. Uncle John always seemed to be smiling through his gentle blue eyes, slightly squinted and his never-ending habit of pulling his watch band from his wrist to the top of his forearm remains a vivid memory. All the uncles and aunts were gathered on the lawn enjoying the day and of course, having a few drinks. Traveler had many cousins that were his age and they decided it was time to experience the wonders of alcohol. The small group quickly found a source of beer down in the basement and discreetly, so they thought, began hauling a few pints out to a place where they could share the cool ale. They were like crows, perching themselves on the limbs of the apple tree south of the homestead. Within a short time, they were not so discreet and their uncles, who were watching from a distance, began laughing, wonderful... no repercussions. Their cousin Roddy was the first casualty as they loaded him into the big black Chrysler station-wagon along with the rest of his family and home they went. Traveler sat quiet in the car on the way home, but the feeling or buzz was well seated.

High School felt like the barn doors had been swung open for the horses to run free in the Spring. He wanted to experience it all and like many, live for the moment.

School dances were the next opportunity to experience shyness & the fear of having to ask a girl to dance and of course the possibility of rejection. Traveler had the solution, and the next dance would be better. His friend Lyle lined up a bottle of Rum from Jumping Jack, the village source of alcohol as they were too young to buy it from the Liquor Store. Lyle & Traveler met at the Fair Grounds, not too far from the High School, to sit under the tree and share the Rum. Laughter kicked in early and they decided to finish the bottle quickly and get to the dance while the Rum's affect was in its' prime. Yes... that worked well, shortly after the first dance Traveler was outside hugging the big Elm tree, feverishly sick and wobbling, the evening was ruined.

Joe drove him home and many times on the way he opened the door to step out, luckily Joe had a quick hand and reeled him back in. Before long he was home and staggering up the stairs, wall to wall. Penny was at the top of the stairs waiting and greeted Traveler with a few sharp words convinced that he was on drugs. He assured her that he was not while falling towards the bathtub, common sense prevailed and he grabbed the shower curtain, quickly wrapped in the plastic as he landed perfectly into the tub. It was going to be difficult to explain that one to Mother. His brothers had already given Penny almost every version of drunkenness, so she was nearing a level of immunity.

Although he was enjoying everything that High School had to offer, good friends, being a player on most school teams and succeeding in class, Traveler's self-esteem was eroding. He would often read the small plaque hanging on the living room wall which read: "Oh God grant that we may be worthy in some small way of the high esteem which we ourselves hold". On the first read or two one might think, what a bunch of egotistical barbarians but it has a deeper meaning, a meaning that Traveler eventually began searching for. His self-doubt was affecting every aspect of his life but did not recognize it or the depth of its power over him. In sports there were moments where he felt exactly in tune and excelled, but many times the mind would fog up and nothing seemed to work in his favor. Self-doubt can be like a poison, slowly taking the life out of you.

It appeared as though God was shining through at times trying to show him all of the potential within him but more often a veil of darkness or clouded feeling would slip over him. It would take a different perception of things to make a change. There was a feeling of frustration, knowing that the potential was within him but that he could not sustain it as the perfection kept eluding him. Traveler was unaware that this little seed of self-doubt had such a hold on him, and he began to shrink inside.

In life there seems to be a few moments or events that remain in one's mind as a vivid memory. There was such an occasion in High School which was a visit from a local Catholic

Priest, Father Cameron. He would conduct a class more as a question-and-answer period, and of course the students were always looking for answers or proof of God's existence, as it appeared there was no real sign other than the Bible's story about the life of Jesus, God's son here on Earth. For sure the priest felt like he was in a room full of non-believers, but he remained confident and finally gave the example that would hit home with a bunch of farm kids. He said in his soft voice "Imagine that you went home tonight and went down to the field and saw bulldozer tracks on the ground, you would automatically without a doubt, say to yourself that a dozer had been working on the farm." All the students agreed to a certain extent but lamented that at least this equipment was real and here with them working in every community and that, for sure was proof. Father Cameron continued by saying that they should look at the miracle of creation, how the dawn of each day brings rise to the Sun which gives another moment of life. Each Spring brings new life to the trees and to the crops seemingly out of nowhere a seed produces a plant and then bears fruit.

He continued talking about the miracle of re-production in livestock, new calves being born each Spring, how is any of that creation possible without a source of power and intelligence that was perhaps beyond their comprehension but nevertheless absolute in Its presence in every aspect of their world.

Once again, the students agreed that at least Father Cameron had cracked the door open to a new understanding of their existence, but they were quick to laugh with him about the fact that they probably wouldn't survive their youth anyways and that they were just going to try and enjoy each moment, sadly enough that was true for one or two students.

Many will say that youth is wasted as they go through those years so naive and little wisdom to guide them along, burning up that precious energy they might lack in their later years of life. There may be some truth to that thought but youth require an enormous amount of energy as self-discovery remains constant each day, who are they, who do they want to become, how do others see them as being. They are determined to cut their own swath and leave their mark; any short falls are only stumbling blocks on their path and their optimism keeps them swinging for a better day tomorrow. As sometimes is the case, the hard knocks in life begin to bring them to their knees and in those moments, reflection prevails which can prompt a little deeper search into that Self-discovery or search for the truth of who they really are and the purpose of being in their experience.

At the age of sixteen and probably before then, Traveler had mastered the art of operating all the equipment that they had on the farm including driving the family car. By this time on the farm there now was a reprieve from the casualties in their family vehicles. Marlene had more sense than to drink and drive which allowed for a second family car. Perfect, it was like Traveler had his own car and by that time he was already familiar with the roads leading to their favorite Bars in Quebec.

Consumption of alcohol and driving seemed to go hand in hand during those early years of being licensed, travelling through the beauty of this rich countryside. An almost endless sea of hayfields, barley and oats swaying under the gentle persuasion of a summer breeze, even the branches of those grand Oak trees and Elms that stood along the winding roads danced in tune without resistance. Many of these moments riding in the 68 Ford Custom were heightened with each sip and the stream of music playing from the AM radio. Although there were legal limits imposed by law it was really at the discretion of the local Police officers whether to enforce these restrictions, mainly because drinking and driving was still an accepted part of the community. Sunday afternoon tours to Quebec seemed perfect, ah… the freedom.

Traveler's first accident was with the same 68 Ford, after a full evening of drinking in Quebec. He had managed to drop all of his friends off at their homes and only had about a ten-minute drive to reach the home place and slip into the sack for a couple of hours before it was time for chores. It was about three o'clock in the morning and his head had already snapped a few times trying to stay awake but finally sleep got the upper hand. It seemed like a second or two that his eyes had closed, but the sound of long grass brushing the bottom of the car was a clear sign that he had left the road. Traveler was wide awake now but no time to react before he hit the four-foot culvert straight in front, which gave him and the Ford quite a lift into the air and over the driveway sliding perfectly between the guide wire and a hydro pole which managed to clip off a mirror and two or three door handles, oh yes… and took the air out of a couple of tires.

The next morning father Sam rode the tractor with Traveler down to Williamstown, there was not much said as his father had been down that road before, not the country road, the one of falling asleep at the wheel. They hooked on the chain and pulled the Ford back out onto the road, changed the flat tires and it was ready for the next journey. A closer look revealed that the frame had been bent up in the front of the car and the back, giving it a new look which his friends soon christened the Rocking Chair.

Their Rocking Chair survived the next year or so and brought them all home safely night after night. Over the next three years Traveler managed to smash another four vehicles, ride in the ambulance and yes… all while under the influence of alcohol. Only by the grace of God and some higher plan in place, did Traveler survive those years and fortunately never affected the life of another in those accidents, there were many others in that area had different outcomes. These accidents and a few others with farm equipment, unknowingly these injuries became collecting points for other hurts and pain throughout his life, memories that became layered one over the other, harboring emotional pain as well as physical, until they were well suppressed at least for a while. At some juncture, the body/mind and emotional energetic body need to heal, so these memories begin to come to the surface to be released. Emotional pain quite often requires forgiveness, not only forgiving someone else but also yourself.

A TIME FOR CHANGE

By the time he was 18 and during that year there was rarely a night that Traveler was not out drinking. He could not get enough of this feeling that he was experiencing with alcohol and the seeming freedom that it brought. There was always a point of awareness being heightened, but with the mind's rationale long subdued by the cool beer, the moment soon turned to drunkenness. Traveler had finished grade twelve but decided in grade thirteen that High School was not for him anymore. He stayed long enough to play a season of football, but not a day longer.

Traveler's father never really commented on his behavior until one night as he was heading out the kitchen door Father Sam stopped him and said, "Traveler, people in the Village are saying that you are turning into an alcoholic." Traveler was quick to toss a comment back at his father saying, "Well that would make most people in this community alcoholics and they should not single him out." The discussion ended there, and he headed out the door. His father's words had struck a nerve and this chapter of his teenage years was nearing an end. It was not the end of his relationship or love affair with alcohol but only the beginning of a different approach, now maybe he was out to prove that he did have some self-worth.

During the year when he was seventeen, he had spent the summer living with brother Hugh and his wife Gloria in New Westminster & worked for Hugh as a laborer building a retirement community. He didn't want to disappoint Hugh who was the foreman on this project, so he worked as hard as humanly possible. The first day on the job, was much to the dismay of his older co-workers who were used to a more relaxed pace. At the end of the day Traveler literally had to slide his hands off the end of the shovel as they had been locked in that position most of the day levelling gravel.

Spending the Summer with Hugh was a great opportunity to begin to know his oldest brother. Traveler's only real memory, other than that special Christmas was when Hugh let him drive his 1958 pitch black Buick convertible with red leather seats and a white ragtop. This drive was only a distance of twenty feet or so in front of the barn just before he and his friends left for the West, British Columbia bound, to make their mark in life. It was a cold January evening when they loaded up the car and headed out, none of them knew what lay ahead, just adventure.

Although some days during that Summer Traveler longed to be back home with his friends and working on the farm, this time spent away was an incredible experience. Waking up to the beauty of the Canadian Rockies that surrounding the city is a view that one could never tire of. Vancouver seemed to be saturated with fresh mountain air, laced with a salty essence from the Pacific Ocean which blended perfectly with the mystic BC fir trees. It is no wonder that Hugh settled in to stay. Hugh and Gloria would often take a drive up the coast to Whistler or into the interior along the Fraser River. Hugh loved to be behind the wheel of his 67 Mustang and it was a real challenge for him to pull over and enjoy the beauty away from the car. Traveler didn't mind just riding and taking in all the raw nature that British Columbia has to offer. He felt that maybe this is where he should spend his life but deep inside the farm was calling him to return.

Summer finally came to an end, so he returned home in September. Being away from home had certainly opened his mind to another world beyond their farming community, a sense of adventure that would be well rooted in his soul. Most of Traveler's friends had finished grade twelve and stepped directly into the workforce either starting a career with the local cheese factory or in another Industry, both opportunities had a good pay scale and pension but that did not hold any attraction for Traveler.

During that Fall he was helping Father Sam out after School, combining corn, filling the Drying equipment, and moving the harvest into Grain Bins. It was also a time to plough the fields and spread manure which was part of the work required to prepare the land for Winter. It was always difficult to predict when the snow would come, but usually the cold settled into stay around the middle of November. A few of Traveler's friends usually helped on the farm over the weekends and of course after the day was done, they would freshen up and head out for an evening fun and drinking beer.

During this time, the farm had a hog barn housing around four hundred pigs. It was never all that pretty entering the barn, normally there was a scurry of mice when Traveler opened the door and always too many to count. Pigs are quiet by nature but only after they have eaten, the noise of a few hundred hungry hogs in unison could certainly get the ears ringing. Lorne, a friend from the village, was usually one of the volunteers to help clean the pig pens which were located on the East farm. All of them could share stories about how cold their homes were during the winter months, but Lorne had the best example. He said that many mornings he would come downstairs to their kitchen only to find that the fire in the wood stove had gone out and the water in the reservoir had frozen. They all had the same sentiment, that leaving the warm bed was always a big decision.

Traveler would be doing chores in one section of the barn while Lorne would be working with the finishing pigs, at least that is what he thought. Traveler went to see if he had completed cleaning the pens only to discover that he had gone outside to sleep on the wagon load of hay. After a few friendly jabs to wake him up, along with some laughter, they returned to finish up their chores.

As the Fall work on the farm was completed, the Winter's air soon brought with it those cold crisp days, a time of year when activity slows down on the farm. By the end of December Traveler and Ernie who was one of Traveler's closest friends, had decided to make the move to Vancouver and perhaps follow in big brother's footsteps. Their desired plan was to find work in the interior of British Columbia surveying or some other adventurous job. Hugh & Gloria had set up part of their basement to accommodate the young Lads. Hugh contacted a few people that he had worked with in the past to help get them started, but B.C. was experiencing a slowdown in most areas of construction and government projects. It was not their plan or dream job, but Ernie and Traveler found work unloading Box cars for a warehousing company not too far from Hugh's home. January and February do not offer up the best of Vancouver and after forty days and forty nights of rain the yearning to return home to the crisp Winters of Ontario and another look at the Sun, was growing.

Traveler spoke a couple of times over the phone with his father and mother about some of the possibilities if he decided to return home. It would be an opportunity to expand and diversify the home farm. It was shaping up to be what he felt could be a continuation of his Parent's dream and the beginning of his.

It was common in Canada for sons and/or daughters to take over the family farm while Parents would stay active on the farm as long as they were physically capable. Eventually perhaps semi-retirement and more time to watch their grandchildren growing up. This had been a cycle in Canada for the past couple of hundred years. In the beginning of the twentieth century ninety eight percent of Canada's population were farmers and as the Country moved through the Industrial age after WWII there was a rapid shift to a point where now less than two and a half percent of the population were living and working on farms.

The seeds were planted, and Traveler would return home to begin planning the future expansion of the farm. Were his spiritual guides busy at work making this life of farming a reality? He was soon to step into a learning experience that would see him through many highs and lows over the next eleven years.

FORK IN THE ROAD

It was in 1974 at nineteen years old where the first fork in the road appeared in the young Traveler's life. These are the moments in our journey where major decisions are made which take us down a new path that is not familiar. If we knew the outcome there is a good chance that we would take a different path but that is the beauty of life, presenting us with the unknown and allowing us to grow as a soul and as a human being. Traveler took this fork in the road asleep at the wheel, no idea of what this expansion of the farm would bring. This would be the first contract with the banking system, something that would eventually begin to control his life. Control can be accomplished when someone has a fear of loss and before signing this contract, Traveler really had no idea how his life was about to change. This contract and a couple of others during the first years of farming brought him in and out of a dark hole which caused stress, emotionally and physically, something he had never felt before.

Traveler's uncle who was a Physician and a Surgeon in their home area often mentioned the word vision. On occasion when he visited the family farm he would ask Traveler, "What do you see when you look at the property, what are the changes." and of course most of Traveler's responses were to do with what he could physically see, not the response Uncle Allan was looking for. Traveler eventually came to understand the word vision but not fully until he began to study all related topics and by then, he was well into his thirties. This ability to form an image in one's mind is a powerful tool, if we learn how to use it to our benefit or not, because a negative image has power as well. The power of thought was not taught in school so it would have to be learned or remembered through Self-discovery. Nearly forty years of Traveler's life passed by before this Universal Law would come to light.

Traveler's father was always a forward thinker and had been involved in the farming community most of his life. He had helped many war veterans establish a new life on farms throughout the area and for a few years taught farming practices to many local farmers during the Winter months.

It seemed like the timing was perfect to expand the family farm, as Canada was experiencing inflationary years during the seventies. Now the banks were making borrowing requirements easier, although the interest costs were still high; something that the family may not have taken into full consideration. His father was building the vision which included having brother Jim, along with his wife MaryJo & their daughter Sara, return home to the farm and be part of the expansion. Jim had the mechanical skills which would be required on the farm and Traveler had a love & passion for animals. It was a perfect plan and they looked at the size of the farm required to sustain three families and what would be the areas of expansion.

Father Sam was already renting additional land from neighboring farms to expand the cash crop business which was mainly for the purpose of growing corn. As new varieties of corn were developed, Eastern Ontario farmers increased the amount of land use for growing this crop. They would expand their land base through lease agreements and improve the farms with systematic tile drainage, the removal of fence lines and fill in the ditches that were no longer required. Bigger equipment would be needed to prepare the land for planting and also for harvesting. Storage facilities, drying equipment and gravity boxes, it was now turning into a large-scale business.

The decision was made to increase the size of the existing hog operation which was at that time thirty-five sows farrow to finish. The farm had an exceptionally good base of Yorkshire breeding stock which could be quickly increased to hundred sows, so they thought. Remember, expansion can sometimes bring pain. They began to draft out a new Swine Facility which would be located on the home farm to house a herd of one thousand hogs along with manure and feed storage and as well include a milling facility for the six hundred tons of rations required to feed the herd annually. With the help of the local Agriculture Office blueprints were completed and the vision began to unfold.

Cash flow projections were completed and if the figures were correct this was going to be a very profitable operation and the realization of everyone's dreams. Hello, hello, hello …There are many unknown factors that come into play with the growth of a company or a farm. The reality began to sink in as everything was in place to create this newly expanded family farm. Over the Summer, loans had been secured in the amount of two hundred and fifty thousand dollars plus. Jim arrived along with his family and a Ryder Truck with all their worldly possessions, family car in tow and moved into the farmhouse (sound familiar, different wagon).

Traveler was excited to have Jim and his family back to live in the community and get to know them as Jim had lived outside Canada for more than fourteen years prior to that time. The farmhouse became their home base for family discussions on how the day was going and experience the evolution of their farm. Most days Jim and Traveler were up at five o'clock in the morning before dawn, mixing concrete to pour another batch of slats that would be required for the dry sow barn.

Within the first few months they were already looking for areas to cut back on construction costs as it appeared, they might be short of funds needed to complete the Swine facility.

Nature's expansion began to push them in a few areas, and she doesn't stop time for anyone. They had about 60 bred gilts living outside ready to help fill the new barn and Winter was coming. The high moisture corn storage needed to be completed in order to bring in the harvest. This new barn, which was key to the expansion was nowhere near completed and yes, Winter was on its way.

Without a doubt the family was not prepared for the chain of events that began to happen as they started to move the herd into the new facility. It was now mid-November so any work outstanding would have to be completed over the Winter months. Looking back perhaps there wasn't anyone in the Swine Industry that could have given them direction as they were breaking new ground in many areas. They didn't have the number of hogs required in the first few months to keep the barn warm during the Winter months, so additional heaters had to be installed. It was difficult not watching the Hydro meter spin as the high costs were adding up. The gilts began to farrow on new concrete that had not cured yet, but one of the costliest lessons was feeding a high moisture ration which should have been an advantage in many ways. Unfortunately, it took two or three years to fully understand the impact that this feed was having on the herd.

When someone is trying to run a profitable hog operation the acceptance of birth and death is hard to handle, especially death. Attachment was beginning to root itself, as there was fear growing about defaulting on the loans. There did not seem to be an issue when the papers were signed, at the age of nineteen Traveler had nothing to lose, so he thought. Now his life was intertwined with other family members and their possessions. Disease and nutrition where the topics of the day as the rate of animal death in the barn was far too high.

Jim and Traveler, with the help of their Father, were maintaining part of the herd at the East Farm while slowly adapting the rest of the animals at the new barn. During the Winter months when the new facility was completed the balance of the herd was moved to their new home. They at least now had the herd under one roof and were able to focus on improving herd health.

There are many times when a salesperson does not get a warm reception, but the boys were in gratitude the day that Ron Davis drove into the farmyard. Ron's company had probably some of the highest quality and best blends of premix for formulating rations in the farming industry. With the help of Ron's nutritional expertise and experienced staff they were able to start eliminating many of the problems that were hampering herd health. They finally got to a point in production where the numbers in the original financial projections were coming to fruition but by then the losses in the barn had caused a higher accumulation of debt, much higher. Perhaps this was the point in time where Jim and Traveler came face to face with stress but did not know its name until many years later. The dream was alive and with the required trait of optimism, which is part of being a farmer, they stayed the course.

Shortly into the expansion of the family farm, Traveler had fallen in love with Fran and within a couple of years they were married. It was while sitting on the bridge late one summer afternoon that he caught a glimpse of her driving by. One moment can change life dramatically, that was one of those life changing moments. They say opposites attract, Fran was a near perfect child growing and Traveler was the other extreme, living on the edge and quite possibly, had not grown up.

Over time the family dream became her dream as she loved country living and the idea of raising a family on the farm. In the first year of marriage, they lived in a 10 X 50` house trailer with walls so thin you could sling a cat through them. The trailer was not really meant to use for Winter accommodations but with a little burlap on the walls and a steady supply of fuel oil, it was home.

Jim and MaryJo by this time had built a new home on the farm and within a year Sam and Penny were living in their dream log home built out of B.C. fir. During that time Traveler and Fran had renovated the farmhouse which soon became home to their son, Rory.

Life seemed to be unfolding perfectly, right on plan, apart from perhaps one small detail which was the burden of debt. It was not going away, and the constant reminder was becoming an anchor around their necks. Many evenings were shared around the kitchen table at Jim and MaryJo's home which was a time for Jim and Traveler to share the day's events with endless laughter. Their Father had picked the right partnership as Jim and Traveler fed off each other's energy with endless humor. Along with this perfect match was the fact that they both loved alcohol and were more than happy to carry on the tradition which was so prevalent in their small community.

Looking back Traveler could see the rationale behind drinking. It is a way to drop all the wasted chatter of the mind and live a moment free, connected to another space where the worries of life could be put aside, only remembering the good moments. In no way is it a long-term solution, but it was what was available at the time. They were not alcoholics, at least Jim would always say that they did not go the meetings (AA), so they were clear.

Winters were long and normally with an abundance of snow so Jim and Traveler would be out on snow mobiles as often as time would permit. One morning after chores Jim and he decided to hook up the toboggan to the back of Jim's Rupp to test out a fresh fall of snow. Traveler is still not sure how he succumbed to this decision perhaps he'll never know but within a few minutes he was hanging on to the ropes on the sides of the toboggan with Jim at the throttle of his 440 Rupp hurdling the wooden rocket across the field at about forty mph. Jim finally stopped at the top of the hill behind their homes, probably to check to see if Traveler was still there. Traveler rolled of the toboggan, looking like the abominable snowman, just the eyes peering through. They were both doubled over with laughter, which really had started shortly after they took flight. Jim was enjoying the event from the comfort of the Rupp, Traveler offered to give Jim a ride on the toboggan but no chance. Traveler rode the toboggan back to the shed but with Jim's word that he'd go a little slower. As the saying goes "If you're not the lead dog the view is always the same." Oh, happy days…

Within a couple of years Jim and Traveler met in the backyard one fine summer morning and agreed on the decision to split up the farming operation. It was the first time in Traveler's life that he had experienced this feeling like he was carrying the earth on his back, he didn't think that his body could have felt any heavier and still be mobile. It is a numbing sensation, holding you almost powerless and no way out.

Within a moment or two the weight began to lift as Jim had been sensing the same as Traveler. They would still be working together as a family but each with their own farm and decisions accordingly. The moment quickly turned into an open discussion as to the best way to divide the land base and assets. The division of the farm was easy, the challenge was in how they would divvy up the heavy load of debt which was slowly sucking the life out of them.

They managed to split up the debt with Jim taking the East farm along with much of the equipment to start cash cropping and Traveler would be his customer for purchasing corn to feed the hog operation. Traveler remained on the home farm with the livestock and so their partnership dissolved but fortunately not their friendship or that of their families. Father Sam by this time had already began working with Ron Davis helping to build the premix business in Eastern Ontario, not something in his original dream but nevertheless, working and helping other farmers was what he enjoyed. Having a couple of sons at home with their families was a good part of a lifelong dream anyway.

Sam shared one day with Traveler, probably over a sip of Scotch that he always wished that he could have the same relationship with his children that Penny had. What he was really trying to say was that he loved them and would like to be able to give his family a hug when the feeling arose. Oh, how the programming of our different cultures and their influence in hindering our true being, which wants to freely express itself. It is a scientific fact that a memory or habit can continue in the DNA of a lineage/family for seven generations, so our responsibility here is to recognize these limiting memories and liberate them. This work, if done in earnest can truly take weight of your heart and bring you peace.

Traveler remembers during those early years hitting his knees in prayer before sliding into bed and praying for some relief, but the occasions in pray were hit and miss and mostly saved for Sunday mass. Early on in Traveler's life prayer seemed directed for better days ahead, and maybe not as much time being spent in gratitude for what they already had. Always the mind pulling them out to a future possibility while missing the blessing of the present moment. That is as true today as it was then.

Once the early hurdles were behind them, the next five or six years on the farm were for the most part a wonderful experience. Fran and Traveler now shared their life with their young children, Charlotte and Rory. Jim and MaryJo had two daughters Sara and Jen who were able to grow up with their cousins next door. The dream was a reality, and the families shared their successes and short falls along the way. Their children were now walking the same farm that their parents had grown up on and the big maple tree on top of the hill remained steady for those ready to make the climb. Traveler looks back at this experience as a gift and one that he will always be grateful for.

Jim and Traveler with the knowledge and assistance of Mr. Kovinich learned the art of roasting a pig on a spit. This newly found method of cooking developed into an occasion for a party in the loafing barn now being used for equipment storage. Jim's mechanical skills soon were at work and fabricated a spit which was driven by an electric motor and family tradition was birthed. The first party planned on the home farm was on the night before the Highland Games in Maxville. Their barn was cleaned up and ready for a couple of wagons which were set up inside to be used as platforms for local musicians and singers. Neighbors were bringing food to share along with the first roast. Jim and Traveler built a fire before chores in the morning and began roasting when the chores were finished. Everything was in place including the kegs of draft beer which they decided to test around nine o'clock that morning, shortly after breakfast. As Gerry O' would always say, "Ah the crack was magic." Gerry was a world class fiddler, born in Ireland and after many accomplishments such as playing for the Queen of England and entertaining a US President or two, he opted for the peaceful life that the village of Martintown offered and became best of friends with Jim. Ah yes, back to the sampling of the keg, as you could imagine by four o'clock in the afternoon more than the pig was cooked, but Jim and Traveler were well seasoned and manage to enjoy a wonderful night of dancing and sharing stories with relatives and friends.

One of the largest roasts and maybe the last held on the farm, was for the School Board trustees who came from across the province of Ontario. Sam was still active in the education of our youth and throughout his life he had completed forty-seven years as a trustee. This meeting for the trustees was held every year but usually in the confines of a five-star Hotel, this would be the first countryside experience. The Coach arrived at the farm, filled to capacity with trustees from across the province. Everything was right on cue; local fiddlers and the most popular musicians were on stage warming up and ready for the evening. There was nothing lacking that evening as the feast was second to none and elegantly served in the barn. It was an occasion that remained for many years as the best experience that the Board members had ever had. Hospitality in this small community and surrounding area remains alive and will likely survive many more generations.

DREAM ON

There are cycles in farming as in every other industry, acting like breath, always flowing ever changing rising and contracting. Traveler had no idea as to how this movement affected or drove the world's economies. Although he tried to educate himself in a night course on how the Stock Market moved and what affected it, there really was not much time to fully understand it and apply the knowledge, at least from the mind's perspective. Life has a way of consuming you if you are not awake to your reality or anyone else's.

In farming these cycles are driven by supply and demand, so the newspaper prints, but for sure there was more to it than that, manipulation, and greed. Mother Earth always provided enough, sometimes an abundance other times more than ample. The cycle in Ontario's Swine Industry usually swung the price up or down in a three-year period but during Traveler's short existence as a hog farmer the cycles were shortened to about every eighteen to twenty-four months. Looking back, it would have been easy to say that he should have been buying futures on the annual feed supply and average out their costs but when one is buried in survival mode options are limited. The focus over a ten-year period was herd health, improvement of the breed lines and hence the production performance.

These cycles were having a dramatic effect on the quality of life more from a standpoint of discussions of money or lack of it. On the higher end of the cycle when hog prices were good Traveler could easily eliminate much of their debt load within six months and if the prices could have held for a few more months he would have been in a position to bear the next down cycle. At this time, cycles were running too close together, and there was not enough time to catch their breath.

Their focus on breeding stock was now paying off and they were raising some of the best pork in Ontario which probably gave them enough pride to hang on through the lean months. Having to leave the farm was thought enough for pain but couple that with eliminating part of his parent's dream and the homestead of Traveler's young family was weighing hard on his heart.

During a short period, Traveler contemplated ending his life a few times, perhaps others have experienced these moments. The fear of death was probably enough to keep the moment at bay coupled with the possibility that he would not be successful on the first attempt kept him grounded and how could one live with that terrible mishap. During the Fall harvest, he would climb the eighty-foot silo each morning to open the hatch to start filling it with corn coming in from the fields. With each step the thought was haunting him. Traveler was weak more from the thoughts than from the climb and he stood there at the top, hanging onto the guard rails like a cat to a wool jacket. His spiritual guides might have brought Traveler´s senses to the view and the beauty that laid before him. This feeling would overtake him, once again as when he was a child, he would close his eyes and feel the breeze, slipping into the bliss. He could hear the honking of the Canadian geese causing his eyes to focus on the flock lifting from the corn field at the back of the farm and far in the distance to the west, the church steeple in St Andrews made clear with the fiery orange rays of the morning sun. Traveler turning to the east, overlooking Jim's farm and the Village of Martintown, history unfolding in silence. Most importantly, another jolt to the senses, the precious young family that Traveler considered leaving behind. After many months he finally came to the realization that he would never do it, never take his life and accepted the fact that he was here for the duration but perhaps one day a life without being a farmer.

Creation is not by accident nor is a soul's journey here, but there is much of it that we are not aware of; by design it is for our individual growth as a soul which ultimately affects the evolution of life in all of God's creation, so our experience can be and is important. When it is time to explore the realization of your Self, again remember the instinct for the Canada goose to migrate, we to are called to journey home. It is to recognize and have the higher essence or Thought Adjuster, integrate within the body, and experience this moment to moment directly to Source in awareness. These seemingly low points in our life can be the moments that help guide the soul to its next awakening and if it is the time, a more focused intention on remembering why one is here and obviously, who or what we are. Freedom becomes of more importance than anything else that a person is experiencing outside of its center or heart space. It is normal to have the mind and body take over the human experience, disconnected from spirit, similar to closing the curtain to stop the sun from shining in, except we are keeping the sun light blocked inside. We are conditioned from a young age until our experience is a function of programming, conditioning, with the great possibility of repeating over and over what is downloaded in our memories. It is through the body and mind that one is able to re-discover Self, but not when the mind is in control of one's experience.

Traveler's crying out to the God he perceived outside of himself, was increasing as the months and years were passing by. The focus was more about gaining freedom again like he had experienced in his youth, freedom at least from this burden of debt, from this heavy heart. The way would come but not yet, there were many adventures that higher-Self still had in plan, would Traveler move into alignment with Creator's Divine idea…

Each day the walk to the hog barn was becoming more and more difficult, Traveler was beginning to feel trapped. He felt so much pride for this herd that had been developed over the past ten years. The peacefulness of the animals every time chores were completed echoed days of his youth feeding cattle, when he could close his eyes and hear the hay being ripped from the feeders and the rhythmic chewing of seventy or eighty head of cattle. Rory and Charlotte were now starting to spend more time with him in the barn and history was repeating itself. Traveler's ego, although somewhat beaten, wanted to maintain a sense of belonging in the community and more importantly, a sense of purpose. Who would he become, he had been a part of this farm and this agricultural community for 29 years of his life…? He was known as the Pigman even since the later years of High School, not such a pretty name but at least it had some definition to it. Once again Mother Earth had hurdled her weight on his back, waiting for a decision before freeing him once again. We all need a push sometimes to make a change, how that pressure is felt is different for each one of us.

On a cold dark day in January of 1985 Traveler walked to the barn early one morning and as every other day completed his chores and listened to the quiet contentment of the animals. This day was different, as the feeling of numbness had become all too prevalent in his being, and he wanted it to end. It was in this moment, with the herd enjoying their meal, Traveler leaned on one of the gates in the finishing barn, looked down the aisle at all that had been accomplished over the past ten years and with a heavy heart, made the decision to leave farming. Once a decision is made, whether it's the right one or not it is like a valve that is opened, and it relieves the pressure that has been building in our being or lifting that heavy feeling from our heart. The earth once again dropped her grip and the mind regained enough clarity to focus on winding down the operation, in preparation for a new experience.

Traveler's decision to leave farming was the beginning of Fran's numb feeling as she loved every aspect of country living and raising their children on the farm. Decisions in life rarely only affect oneself or yourself, those new directions reach out to touch many. Traveler made the trek across the property to his parent's home to share his decision with them and as expected his father's mind was heading in a direction of salvaging the farm, but Traveler was far beyond that thought as he had lived with it for far too long. Juggling the financing and looking at other options, those were behind him. In a short time, they were as always, supportive of his decision and a different life for Traveler was about to begin.

Ron Davis stepped into the family's life once again and asked the question if Traveler would be interested in becoming a salesman for his company and help to build his premix business with more focus on swine operations. Traveler had completed a few feed trials in his herd for Ron, during the last few years and certainly had the belief in Ron's product and in his nutritional staff. Traveler wasn't sure if people were born with sales genes in their blood, but it is a profession that could be learned. Ron's offer which included a vehicle and training in his production plant on other products seemed like it would be the best transition from farming to the outside world. A few weeks of training along with the keys to a company truck and the new career began to come to life.

Traveler was fortunate enough to spend a month or so with father Sam driving throughout the countryside of Eastern

Ontario, much of which he had never seen before. Each new day consisted of visiting farmers to gather feed samples which would be labeled and couriered to the Lab from the Berwick Plant. It was a great experience learning firsthand his father's knowledge on all aspects of farming and as well on his outlook about life. Traveler became more knowledgeable on dairy farming something that he was not really educated on. There are complexities to properly feeding a herd of milking cows and this information could only be learned through time and experience.

Traveler had the pleasure of walking through many dairy barns and sharing in the farmer's pride of a lifetime of herd improvement and good management. It is quite a pleasurable experience to see fifty Holstein cows, groomed and standing on a thick bed of straw. Some of the best dairy cows are raised in Eastern Ontario and continue to be shipped for breeding stock to many countries around the world. There was a feeling of satisfaction being able to be a part of this community of farmers, even indirectly.

It was now time to venture out on his own and focus more attention to hog farms spread across the countryside from the town of Pembroke East to the Quebec border. Traveler was given some of his father's existing customers to look after which included many dairy farmers who he had known most of his life, this was truly a gift to work with neighbors and good acquaintances.

Ron was a gifted salesman and spent time and resources with each salesperson to ensure that they were working as efficiently and productively as possible. Salespeople have an opportunity to share in the rewards of a company with no limits on their earning potential. Their only limitation was in self-development, an area Traveler began to understand as Ron shared stories of his younger days in sales. He had been the top salesman in a company early on in his career and his ego felt that there was no room for improvement but finally he conceded long enough to listen to an expert in self-development. Ron was full of skepticism but remained open minded as a student and soon began to experience a huge increase in his sales achievements. He understood the power of self-development and tried to instill this possibility of greatness within each one of his salespeople.

Now motivational talks are wonderful, but they are similar to putting gas in your car it is not long before more is required. In order to increase sales, you must call on new prospects something that rooted up every weakness in Traveler's body. Remember the problem he had walking back from communion, nothing had changed, at least not yet.

He would recall a story told by his neighbor Stuart and his greeting for a salesperson making such a call to the farm. Stuart leaned in the window of this person's car and went through the usual courtesies of good-day and then asked if he had reverse in his car which the man acknowledged with a nod and a yes. Stuart continued with, "Good, then back your **?!!?* car all the way to the road (a mere half mile away) and get out of here." Just the kind of thoughts Traveler needed to assist him in getting over any personal hurdles when faced with a cold call.

Traveler enjoyed almost every aspect of working with farmers and their livestock. There were so many satisfying moments when herd health & production began to improve, and the owner's profitability would increase. There was from time to time, the addition of a new customer, along with their first order which undoubtably seemed to give him strength to try and repeat the process. This small achievement helped but similar to any type of motivation it can be short lived. One beautiful sunny day he was heading down the road to a new prospect for his first call of the day. Traveler soon found himself pulled over in the ditch sitting in the truck full of self-doubt and allowing the mind to take him on a trip full of questions. Did he really need this job or is there something easier that he could be doing, and after a long session of inner chatter he decided not to allow the lack of self-esteem to cripple him, at least not today and continued on to the farm where he was greeted with a friendly smile. Doubt and fear can paralyze us if we let it, our choice can be to recognize it for the energy that it is and rise above it.

Life's journey is different for each one and many situations that are encountered along the way seem insurmountable, what may be killing one person inside might be a non-issue for another, but most people have their hurdles to cross over. It is a choice to push forward and overcome our worst enemy which truly is memory based, emotional and physical. This fear within, the feeling of not being good enough can make us succumb to those negative energies and shrink inside. It is said that to live in fear is to die a death every step of the way, whereas when you overcome fear, you die only one death. A death of all the misunderstood memories from this lifetime and past, can be the start of living in the present, the start of lifting the weight. When we consciously begin to work at removing this pain and suffering that has accumulated over time, it enables this inner light to shine through and we can begin to experience this peaceful state of being that has always been our true nature.

Traveler continued working for Ron for two and a half years traveling the roads and continuing to build a customer base. Although ever so slowly he was beginning to remove some inner-doubt and feel a sense of accomplishment that was rooting itself within. Ron felt that Traveler was ready for the next level of sales training and had planned to send him to Syracuse for a few days, an experience that he truly was looking forward to.

Throughout these years they were still gathering around the kitchen table at Jim and MaryJo's, to share the activities of the week over a jar or two. They would share the memories of their youth and Jim often laughed as he would say," I'm the pretty one Mary". Often, they were treated to a slice or maybe two of

MaryJo's delicious carrot cake after supper. Traveler could safely say that although he had sampled many similar cakes, none could compare. It was a time where their families seemed to be progressing quite well and enjoying raising their children, but Life was about to present another fork in the road.

Jim through a friend of his mentioned the fact that a local company was looking for an Equipment Manager and maybe he should inquire about the position. Within a few days Traveler was sitting in an interview with the Manager of Operations and going over the responsibility that the new position held. There were two major reasons for his interest in the position, one being an additional ten thousand per year in salary which included a company vehicle and the fact that he would only be commuting to the city which was only twenty minutes away from home. At last, a decision in his life that came without stress, one that felt right for Traveler and his family.

Another change was coming, motivation of some sort always plays a part, it can be from a point of pain or for economic increase which is usually a nice choice. In either case, one is stepping into the unknown, a new environment, new people, and different energies. The more aware a person is the easier the transition is. Traveler was not quite awake yet, taking the fork in the road while asleep at the wheel.

COUNTRYSIDE TO THE CITY

Although Traveler was familiar with most equipment that was used for farming and for general construction, there was much to learn in the mechanical/electrical field. His work was to manage the Equipment Division which was new for this company. In their efforts to become more efficient, the purpose was to house an accurate inventory of all equipment that would be required on the jobsites. At times, the Equipment Division would supply tools and equipment for between three hundred and six hundred trades people. The jobsites were from Napanee to the Quebec border and many times in remote areas of Ontario and Quebec. Traveler soon began to realize the depth of this task that he had been hired for and was excited to get started.

This newly renovated building with an office, a mechanics area for vehicle and heavy equipment repair along with a storage area was now complete. As jobs were completed the idea was to bring all equipment in for servicing and add it to the company's inventory list. Staff were hired to repair and maintain equipment as well as catalogue new and existing tools.

The idea was excellent but as is the case many times in life, there was a lack of communication with the people out on the jobsites. During the past twenty years or so each job superintendent was responsible for buying equipment for each project and usually tried to maintain these tools from one site to the next. Here was one area where the company was trying to become more efficient as many of the tools were either lost or stolen, which mounted up to a significant loss of profit for the company. Hence the new Equipment Division would track all purchases, tag tools & equipment and act as a rental depot for each jobsite. Seemed like a great idea.

Traveler's training was more of here are the keys to the building and a short walk around to familiarize him with the layout. There was an introduction to a few key people in the company, but he was ill prepared for the uproar that was about to begin. Traveler was given a strict mandate to the effect that no equipment would leave the building unless it was accompanied with a rental agreement and a job number. That seemed simple enough, but it became clear that it was almost impossible, at least in the first couple of months.

His first encounter was with Guy one of the job superintendents who had been with the company probably since day one. He stood at the counter and began shouting words that were not fit for a dog let alone another human. Traveler was sure that Guy had not read the book, "How to Win Friends & Influence People". Through a number of these heated discussions and a loosening up of policies for personal use, the Equipment Division slowly began to be accepted and an easier way to prepare for each new project. Many of these irate managers became Traveler's friends and best allies which are many times required in dealing with the politics of this industry.

Their inventory continued to grow as they completed onsite tagging of tools along with the returns from completed jobs. The equipment division was taking on a life of its' own and soon it required a secretary, a second mechanic and two full-time employees preparing equipment orders for the ongoing jobsites. It was becoming a challenge to keep up with the growth and demand.

All company vehicles were tracked under their inventory along with service records. The first estimates that they had received was around fifty vehicles which soon grew to over eighty as people began to bring their vehicles in for service. Traveler was continually sourcing out suppliers for equipment replacement. Much of the equipment had lived through its cycle of life and newer machinery, as well as tools were added to the inventory.

Allan, who had worked with Traveler on the farm was now working alongside him once again and as well Gerry a family friend. Allan's father, Donald had worked on the farm from time to time, you could say that their families were like family. Traveler has many fond memories of him, one was when they were riding on the tractor with Donald standing on the draw bar heading towards the river. While they bounced up and down on the farm lane Donald reached back and pulled out a piece of wire from his back. Donald had been hit with shrapnel during a battle in WWII and the mesh was implanted to support his back.

Donald was always willing to share a story sitting, sometimes on the tailgate of his 58 Chevrolet Apache pickup while rolling a fresh Players cigarette with one hand. Traveler could still hear the snap from the cover of his Zippo lighter as he slipped it back into his pocket. Where did life change and take a turn? It all seemed so simple when he was growing up on the family farm, everybody just flowed with the day, and in that flow were moments just to share their experience.

Traveler and the small group managed to keep up with the demand for equipment on the jobsites. Their original schedule was seven o'clock in the morning until four o'clock in the afternoon. Before too long their jobs had now turned into late nights and working on Saturday mornings to complete their work. They enjoyed each other's company which helped to maintain a good work environment. Part of a manager's role is to develop a good team of people that complement each other and help support the efforts of all. If there is a weak link in the group, it has to be addressed. Sometimes a discussion with a fellow worker can help to find the source of the problem but if over time the problem persists then the weak link must be removed. Traveler had never had the unpleasant task of firing anyone and as the inevitable moment drew nearer so did the anxiety growing within him. He prolonged it for many days until he was starting to feel sick, so finally he drummed up enough courage and called their secretary into the office. Traveler shared the reasons for his decision in a calm manner that day, but it quickly became clear that the moment did not go well. She left the office crying and went home only to return in less than a half an hour with her boyfriend who was looking to set things straight, fortunately he left after only sharing a few harsh words. Communication skills help but there is no way of knowing how the message will be received.

Traveler was beginning to see a different world and he was uncertain if anyone was cut out for the dog-eat-dog way of etching out a living. In time Traveler would come to realize a grander plan in life but for the moment he accepted that employee replacement was a necessity when all other efforts fail. Within a month or so this individual (Secretary) was back on track in her life as she entered a new career path which was much more rewarding than working at the Tool Crib. Each of these experiences helped Traveler to see that once again the dark moment which could present a fork in the road of life, can be a turning point towards something better.

Traveler was now at a place in his daily routine where it was becoming more difficult to maintain this pace of long hours week after week. He was working at his desk one morning and found himself swaying in his chair from one side of the desk to the other, like a mentally challenged horse standing in a stall. The task was not that difficult, only trying to decide which stack of paper to pick up. He kind of laughed at himself and wandered what was that about...? He had been experiencing a lot of pain in his joints but thought maybe it was from the dampness coming up from the concrete floors. It was time to investigate, and he made an appointment with a Doctor in Ottawa at the Sports Clinic, he had to start somewhere.

After the usual tests and x-rays it was time for a discussion with the Doctor. He said that everything looked fine except for a small piece of cartilage floating around in Traveler's left knee, probably from football or a car accident but no cause for pain. He asked about Traveler's work and his daily routine which he explained in detail. The Doctor kind of laughed and asked if he had ever heard of stress and explained the many ways that it can affect your body & mind and ultimately your health. Traveler remembered Jim and himself coming face to face with stress but was not aware of the way it could affect your health. He drove home relieved in one sense but at that moment he also vowed that somehow, he would never knowingly let stress back into his life.

Traveler had a little exercise that he used when he was farming, it was to energize his body. He would sit or lay down and bring each limb into stillness along with the trunk of his body then finally the neck and head. Once that was accomplished then he would count slowly to twenty and relax with his eyes closed. When he felt it was time to awake, he would then count backwards from twenty to zero and open his eyes. This exercise usually lasted ten to fifteen minutes and it was amazing how it cleared the mind and energized him for the rest of the day. Traveler still had not heard about meditation or connecting to source, yet it had been right at the tip of his nose.

Samuel McLeod

The Doctor had mentioned a few things about diet and Traveler became a little more conscious of what he was eating. A few subtle changes and just the fact that he could now recognize the symptoms of stress helped him to eventually clear it from his life. The workload did not slow down but each time he felt himself beginning to sway or lose control he would stop and become centered once again.

Life seems to have a way of teaching us with lessons that many times the call to learn will surface through our health whether it is mentally, emotionally, or physically. As the level of awareness continues to increase perhaps one recognizes these subtle signals early and make a few changes in their life. Extremes in life, if continued for long will throw the experience out of balance. Traveler remembers a story shared by Chloe Ann who had her massage therapy office in small city not too far from his home. She said that as a teenager she was usually out partying most nights, seems normal, but during those years many high school kids lost their lives in car accidents. Chloe's father was very aware of these events as he was a doctor in the community. One morning after a long night she stumbled downstairs to greet the day, there she met her father waiting for a chat. He was not hard on Chloe Ann but calmly said to her that life needs to be lived in balance, too much of a good thing can begin to affect your life in an adverse way. She never forgot that moment and has been aware of maintaining balance in her life ever since. Chloe Ann works most every day but always schedules time off so that she can enjoy an afternoon at home riding her horse or spending time with her family on the farm.

It was the eighties, and that decade was now coming to an end and the vibrant economy that Canada had been experiencing over the better part of 20 years was about to enter a period of adjustment. Traveler understood a bit about the short cycles in farming but was unaware of the longer cycles in a country's economy and even less on what was the cause. Most of the Canadian population along with businesses were enjoying these inflationary years and the accumulation of material things for their enjoyment of life.

At first, companies thought that it would only be short term and tried to keep things status quo but that was short lived as overhead costs began to cut into company reserves. Traveler's company did not escape this downturn either and as projects were completed equipment was returning to the shop until they were short of space. There were very few new projects being awarded to the company and lay-offs were becoming a weekly event. Bitterness was becoming common as many employees who had been with the company for the past fifteen to twenty years felt that it was unfair after being so loyal. Somehow, they had a feeling of security with the company and did not anticipate having to change. There is no security in any company, all are susceptible to change and as it was becoming the constant, many people from that point on would experience a career change perhaps four or five different times during their working life.

Eventually, as the axe continued to swing within Traveler's company, it finally made its way to the office door, offering another fork in the road, and it was decision time again. Remember the political ties within the company, well Traveler's connections were not quite far enough up the ladder to escape the affects. A favor was being called in and Traveler was being replaced by one of the site managers who was now being displaced from his position. It seems like the flow is always down the chain of command. Traveler knew inside that he had given this position his best effort and the division's performance had shown it on the bottom line of the company's ledger. The ole ego took a hit, but it would not be the last one.

Traveler was more adept to change than most and still maintained optimism in his soul, grown from his days of farming. It was made clear that the change was not because of performance or work ethics and for that effort the company was willing to pay for his time & training in any trade related to the mechanical or electrical industry. The offer was more than fair and one that he was grateful for.

After some consideration he chose to attend the Crane Operators course in Toronto partly because he enjoyed working with equipment. He was soon registered and began classes which required six weeks to complete and his mandatory seat time as it is called would be completed with the company. Marlene and Don were kind enough to open up their home for his stay and he commuted from Oshawa to Toronto daily. It was not long into the first week that Traveler firmly decided that living in a large city fighting traffic morning and night would not be a life for him and was looking forward to returning home.

His first week in class was a little overwhelming as the brain seemed to ache from retrieval of things learned in High School along with new knowledge required to operate a crane or boom truck safely. He was training each day on different boom trucks as this was the license that he wanted to obtain. One of the Instructors was a constant reminder of the safety required while working around this equipment. His forehead looked like an axe had split it, he had the unpleasant experience of a load chain snapping and the hook came barreling over the truck to catch him right between the eyes. Not pretty. Traveler began to enjoy every aspect of the course and almost a year later he received a call to inform him that he had earned the Highest Achievement Award for the class. Sometimes it is the little accomplishments in life that give a person strength to take on the next challenge that they are faced with.

Traveler's career as a boom-truck operator was short lived as the effects of a slowing economy continued to hamper stability in the work force. Yes, it was time for another decision in his life, an event that seemed to be coming more often. We can embrace the fork in the road during our life as it represents an opportunity to grow. Creator experiences Life through us, we are co-creating and evolving, not only for ourselves but for humanity and all other forms of life throughout creation.

RESTAURANT – TOUGH SCHOOL

It was during the summer of 1989 when Traveler began to ponder on a new career. They had now completed building their second home east of the village. Their first home, after leaving the farm, was built on a wooded lot overlooking some of the richest farmland to the south, the winding Raisin River, and on a clear day the Adirondack Mountains. Real Estate prices had been rising for a few years, so the decision was made to sell their home and build on the other side of the road, same view but with more land.

The building of these two homes had opened Traveler's mind, as he remembered his uncle's thoughts about vision. There is something magic about home construction as you can either select a design or create one which was the case in their second home. An aroma of rich earth fills your senses as the Excavator begins to dig the foundation, nothing is more rewarding than watching the changes each day during construction until only the landscaping remains to complete. Traveler was slowly beginning to realize the power of thought at least in its positive sense. If only this knowledge had been taught in school how different the world might be. The system seemed to be designed to consume life with jobs and family responsibilities and did not leave much room to explore the creative potential of thought, too busy making a living to make a life. Oh, the waking up can be ever so slow but not the first experience here asleep at the wheel.

Many times, in life, opportunities come along, and decisions are required to be made quickly at least we think so. Upon looking back, Traveler would say that opportunities are forever presenting themselves we just need to be prepared to accept them or let them go by and wait for the next one, there is no shortage in this ever expanding Creation. The controlling society of this world keeps many people in an action/re-action type of experience, not much chance of peace in there. Whatever it takes to liberate the soul and live in that peace within, is worth the effort.

Housing prices had reached their peak in the real estate cycle, not something that Traveler was aware of, but the timing allowed them to take advantage of the equity that was in their home. Through their friend, they were given an opportunity to purchase a Restaurant located in the nearby city. Mickey was respected businessperson so there was a level of confidence in this purchase/sale. Traveler and Fran looked at the cash-flow generated by the Restaurant which had been in business for almost ten years. Traveler had learned to cook at the age of fifteen when Penny decided she wanted a new challenge in her life, away from the farm, and worked in the city for about a year. His father denied having any cooking skills, so Traveler soon became the cook-bottle washer so to speak. He loved to cook, he had business experience and their family were well known in the area, perfect where do they sign. Hello, hello, hello… Here is a point in life well remembered and the word to describe it is non-disclosure in every sense of the word.

Traveler knew nothing about the Restaurant business which might have been his first clue to slow down on the decision to buy one. Statistics showed that after five years in business ninety five percent of all restaurants went out of business having suffered losses or gone bankrupt. Thanks for the tip but Traveler had good work ethics and really, it could not be any more difficult than farming. Oh yes it could... He still had optimism flowing through him and once again, the cash-flow looked extremely attractive. He had experience in management and in working with employees. The blinders were firmly in place, and he took a left in the fork on the road.

The bank was willing to provide bridge financing and before the paint was dry on their new home it was up for sale. This home was beautiful as was the stunning view from the living room and dining room. It had a natural spring located on the hill that could supply a small village, fifty acres of prime land which with the right project could have supported the family. This was a time when strawberry and raspberry farms were being developed as the desire for people in the city wanting to go out for a drive and pick their own produce. Traveler still has some residual fear of farming, never even crossed his mind. Their intention was to keep the Restaurant for five years and then sell it, so when the moment came, they could always find another piece of land and build again.

By October 1st Traveler had a little training under his belt and the keys to their Restaurant in hand. The Diner opened officially at six o'clock in the morning, but the first customers usually started arriving at five thirty and from that point on the flow of people did not stop until closing at two o'clock in the afternoon. He was getting up at four o'clock in the morning in order to arrive at the Diner by five o'clock and start the prep work along with their main cook. He could not have imagined the amount of work involved in running a Restaurant, but it soon became clear.

Within the first few days, perhaps the first day, he knew that he had bit off more than he could chew but he figured that he would adapt to the pace at some point. Traveler lost 10 lbs. in the first month partly from the fact that they were so busy that there was little time to eat. Traveler had mentioned something about he was not going to allow any stress back into his life, but the little doll had arrived for a visit and this time she had her suitcase packed preparing for a five-year stay. What could possibly be wrong, the Diner was extremely busy, and the cash-flow was there. Well, here he was in a mental space, more like a predicament that he vowed he would never return to and that was, the burden of excessive debt. They were carrying over $250,000 of debt and would be until their house sold. They had put the family's home equity on the line and had that thought every morning as he crawled out of bed in darkness to prepare for another grueling day. There were closing costs that absorbed profits for the first few months but finally with the help of Divinity their house sold and by that time Traveler was adapting to the pace.

Here is a little bleep about non-disclosure. The friend did not have a clue about restaurants, fair enough neither did Traveler. The asking price was one hundred thousand but after the first meeting with the owners he suggested that we should bump the offer up to one hundred and fifty thousand as there was another interested party. Maybe so, but there could not have been another idiot in the same city, there was only room for one in this deal. His friend forgot to mention that the owners rarely took a day off, never gave the staff a break to eat or rest. That meant extra staff and more costs, to permit each employee at least one break during the day. Five years commitment eh, soon be over… In all fairness, Traveler had the final say concerning this fork in the road, so the purchase could have been delayed a bit to get all the facts, which usually come out with time.

Now it was time to build a team of people that Traveler felt comfortable with and could make their workplace an enjoyable experience. The Diner required three waitresses, two cooks, with Traveler being one of them and two dishwashers to handle the flow of hungry customers each day. It was time to make an adjustment in the team and the first casualty was one of their best waitresses although they all worked exceptionally hard. Once again that went over well and he received a couple of calls long after he was horizontal for the night, to share her thoughts. It took a little over a year to finally have a group of people working with at the restaurant that he thoroughly enjoyed being with.

During their first year in business there was a toll on Traveler's health, as employees were replaced and new ones were trained, this process sometimes meant that he would have to work weeks without a day off to rest. They had moved into the city that year which gave Traveler an extra twenty minutes of sleep each day, ah… it is the little things in life. It seemed like they had just walked in the front door of their new city home and out the back one. Fran had become a country girl, wanting to raise their family there, so the decision was made to build another house near the golf course at the city's edge. This time Traveler would over-see the construction of their new home, purchase material, line up the trades etc. The Diner closed at two o'clock in the afternoon that should allow lots of free time to build a house. Where was the rationale in this hair brain idea, oh maybe it was the thought of repeating an increase in equity, which they were blessed with on their first two homes. Not awake yet…They were not aware of the Real Estate cycle that was about ready to bust or in fact already had begun its downturn. How could Traveler have known, there was no time to study trends only time to try and keep ahead of the expenses. He loved building homes and if not for the stress of debt it probably energized him. Again, the little Diner had to carry the burden of bridge financing, such a fancy term, while their home was being built. The Diner never really had a chance to come up for air, neither did Traveler.

The ego always likes to be busy and maintain a sense of purpose or more accurately, control and it was safe to say that

Traveler was busy. The moment had arrived, the scent of fresh earth being piled up as the Excavator began to dig a hole for the foundation. Any time that he caught the scent of earth being turned over, usually when a farmer was ploughing the field, it immediately brought him back to the farm and a desire to return to that way of life. One thing about debt is that it gets you out of bed in the morning and keeps you swinging during the day to make sure that you could keep up with your commitments. There must be a better way to spend your efforts than working for the bank.

The house was completed a few months later and the family were able to settle into a more normal pace and routine in their life. A wonderful group of employees, more like friends were now in place at the Diner and the workplace was once again an enjoyable environment. Penny had taken over as the Pastry Chef and was preparing her famous pies for customers at the Diner. The Restaurant was becoming more of a family atmosphere, an enjoyable experience for customers. Traveler would have to say that if it was not for the grueling schedule of a Restaurant, he would have considered keeping the business longer than 5 years. The family had an immense amount of affection for the staff and shared in their lives.

At this juncture in Traveler's life, all looked pretty normal, he had a wonderful family along with a beautiful home on the Golf Course and a Restaurant that was providing a comfortable lifestyle. Rory was working at the Golf Course which helped him to develop good work ethics and within a short period of time he became an above average player. On the surface Traveler had a near perfect life with only one underlying factor which was, could he keep up the pace. Every morning when he crawled out of bed his first thought was to slip back in. He had become accustomed to getting up early on the farm as his Father never wanted the Sun to burn a hole in their back, but the pace at the Restaurant was deteriorating his health and he couldn't regain his strength.

Traveler always maintained a relationship with God, but it was probably during this moment in time that they talked a little more often, well… maybe Creator was listening. Traveler was looking for relief, a lottery perhaps, seldom does the change come as one would like it or on any kind of schedule. Higher Self has an adventure in plan that sends the soul out to experience, neither one of them sends the plan along to this plane.

One weekend at the Diner brought about the beginning of a major shift in Traveler's life, another fork in the road, one that has continued to this day and will continue until this lifetime is complete. He had come to know or at least recognize many customers but there were many that he did not know. Even though the kitchen area was open to the seating area in the Diner most days were spent spinning in circles trying to keep up with the orders. By this time Fran had opted for job sharing at her work and was now helping at the Diner a few days a week.

A customer had given Fran a cassette tape and asked her if Traveler would take the time to listen to it and let her know his thoughts concerning the information.

Uncle Allan had talked about success in life as being attained through the efforts of others that work for you in your own business. Traveler should have been right on track with the Diner but perhaps unknowingly he was looking for a better way. This young woman asked if she could pick the tape up in a few days giving him lots of time to listen to a twenty-minute tape. He tried every night for almost a week but could never finish it before falling asleep. The Diner closed at 2:00 o'clock in the afternoon but there was usually maintenance to do after closing along with banking, laundry and picking up supplies. By the time the family finished supper and the rest of their daily chores it was almost 9:00 o'clock at night and time for bed. This patient woman could not understand why it was taking Traveler so long. He finally listened to the full 20 minutes and the concept seemed to make perfect sense, He was physically tired, but open to finding for a better way.

A meeting was arranged for the following week with a person who was pursuing this business concept and someone who had experience. Traveler met him at the Diner after closing and Syl began to spin the dream, Traveler felt that there was not any area of their discussion that he did not agree with. When Syl finished with his presentation he mentioned that the company he was affiliated with was the Amway Corporation. It didn't send a chill down Traveler's back because Penny had used these products back in the 60's and often spoke about their good quality.

A short story here; one of the neighboring farmers, back in the 60s was selling Amway products, he arrived at the family farm and is the norm Penny invited him into their home. Traveler happened to be at the house that day, so he was a witness as well as a participant. The farmer had a strong French accent so try to imagine that. He started to sell Penny on the benefits of the laundry soap, somewhere in there he slipped in the fact that it would actually remove stains out of your underwear. Traveler, who was about eight or nine years old at the time, was sitting at the bottom of the steps leading upstairs and in hearing this he let out a grunt and headed upstairs laughing out of control, what he hadn't counted on was Penny coming right on his heels as she was laughing beyond control herself and looking to hide until she could gain some composure. Traveler and Penny were there quite a while, not able to stop laughing, it was inevitable that Penny would have to return alone to finish off listening to the sales pitch, what more could be said, it was an effective product...

Traveler took another tape home and tried to figure out where he would find the time to add this into his life. As is most common in choices made, it is not the effort that we look at, it is the reward and for Traveler it was trying to create a sustainable cash-flow before his body was worn out. He felt like he would not have enough energy to accomplish what he wanted in is his life. Where to sign and what is the quickest way to get started, the decision was made.

With the possibility of financial freedom fully renewed in his life this feeling brought with it a new source of energy, yes… no idea what he was getting into. He quickly became a student of network marketing and for the first time in his life he began to read, at least more than the news. The last and probably the only book that he had ever really completed was the Hardy Boys.

Amway had an endless supply of motivational tapes and books which he began to devour. From the time he stepped into his Astro Van in the morning heading for the Diner until he went to bed at night he was listening to tapes. He quickly developed the thought if they can do it so can I. Non-disclosure comes to mind… Traveler was motivated by the fact that he wanted to get out of debt and the constant feed of tapes and books kept his motivation at its peak. This customer along with Syl had cracked open a door in Traveler's life that sent him down a path of no return, that fork in the road.

Within a short period of time Syl was back sitting in the Diner spinning the dream with Joey. Traveler had known Joey only briefly as he had worked with his relatives on the farm and for the same company that his father had. Joey was a little more hesitant than Traveler was but looked at Traveler's seemingly successful life with the Diner and home on the golf course and decided that it was worth the pursuit. They were on the roads most nights either holding meetings or attending up-line functions. Many times, the people that they met had illusions of success that were similar to Traveler's, as they had accumulated debt while pursuing their dream.

One of their most grueling trips was to the Dome in Atlanta. They left after work, with Sylvain at the wheel. Fortunately, there were enough drivers to complete the 20-hour trip and Traveler was able to sleep most of the way. There were always great speakers from ex-football stars to comedians. In Atlanta ex-President Bush Sr. spoke about family values, it was a memorable time, seem to fit into life and all that they were doing or trying to do.

Amway seemed a lot like AA, most gatherings had a spiritual content or more likely religious, to help get them fired up, in the ole build the business mode. Although Traveler was not comfortable with many aspects of these functions, he figured that perhaps it was just his own self-doubt and low self-esteem that would not allow him to fully participate.

Jack and Effie were the up-line diamonds for this group function held in Pennsylvania. One evening at the close of this event, Effie asked if anyone would like to come to the stage and accept Jesus into their life. Traveler was nearing the point of surrender, white flag in hand, and although he always felt a relationship with God and Jesus, they were still somewhere out there. Traveler was feeling weary but stood in line and shortly after it was his turn to embrace Effie. Effie was a firecracker, full of energy but she was taking this moment seriously. She asked Traveler if he was ready to accept Jesus into his life and then gave him a long heart-felt hug. Traveler felt like someone was standing on his chest, there was a lot of pressure in his heart, something distinct. It was perhaps a moment that began a deeper search into what had happened, spiritual growth, maybe…

Joey and Traveler along with another person from Montreal who was in Sylvain's organization were on the road again and heading for Kentucky, if there was a function they were there. Life has a way of catching up with you at times and can bring you to your knees on the ground but eventually one begins to realize that all moments are gifts from our Source. It was shortly after mid-morning when they arrived, the Explorer was parked on the street across from a baseball field, and they stepped out to greet the day. A beautiful day it was, clear blue skies with only a few snow-white clouds floating aimlessly. Traveler was standing there on the street, alone with his thoughts of surrendering his life to God. What did that mean, how should he approach this Creator, He seemed so distant… Traveler had a fair bit of fear circling around like the Chicken Hawk in cartoons, maybe he would have to become a Priest or a man of the cloth which he really wasn't prepared to do. Finally, he decided that he would accept the outcome as he could not do it on his own anymore. He leaned back on the hood of the truck and looked up at the blue skies, with full conviction that that is where God resided and perhaps Jesus was just down the road in another Pueblo, but in that moment, Traveler surrendered his Life to Him. He wasn't hit by lightning as happens so often in the Hollywood movies, but it was the beginning of a life with more awareness and a flow of information through Self, experiences and books that began to transform Traveler's thoughts and feelings about his existence here and beyond. He was determined to find the Truth and that became the burning fire within, all else was secondary.

Fortunately, the little Diner had a significant enough cash-flow to sustain the out-flow of thousands of dollars in motivational material and travel. Joey and Traveler became best friends over the years and many times laughed at the amount of effort and resources that were being spent. They often said that their education was expensive but something that could not be bought. If one is steadfast in his goal of finding the Truth during his lifetime, he will be given all the necessary resources and knowledge to reach that point. He will be given the circumstances to guide him, absolute trust in your Source is needed, trust in your-Self and loyalty to your Self.

Traveler's stamina was becoming less & less as each year passed so he and Fran decided to sell their home by the golf course and move back into the city. The real estate market was still in a down cycle and homes in the $250,000 price range had dropped as much as $50,000 in value. They were blessed that their home was located near the course which helped to maintain a higher value. They moved to a smaller home and lowered their debt substantially and this allowed a little breathing room to live.

It was in the fall of 1994 just before Halloween when Traveler developed a cough which quickly turned into pneumonia. His body's immune system had hit bottom and he could not stop shaking from being cold. He was on antibiotics at home for one week trying to get better so that he could return to work at the Diner. On Sunday of that week, he decided that some fresh air might help, and they crossed over the border to the United States for breakfast, that went well, he couldn't stop shaking while he was eating, no control of the body. Monday morning Penny was at the door to take Traveler to the Hospital and by that time he was ready. After the tests were completed, the young Doctor stood at the bedside and said, "You're not doing too well, are you." He looked like he had a little fear mixed with a hint of confidence but in this moment, Traveler was helpless, just do what you must do. They alternated antibiotics for a period of one week in the Hospital to see if they could knock this virus as his white blood cells were off the chart. It is never a good thing to hand your health over to someone, but if you live through it is a great opportunity to take it back. After one week he gained a little strength and went home to recover completely.

Traveler had never really been ill any longer than a day or two in his entire life and he told Fran that he should be able to return to the Diner in another day or so. She laughed and told him that he would be fortunate if he could return in 6 months. Traveler began to believe her after a few weeks as afternoon naps had become a daily routine just to build up enough energy to walk around the house. He could not climb up five or six steps without laying down to rest, laughing to himself that he was so weak. They were blessed to have staff in the Diner that were honest and had good work ethics. With Fran's extra effort and the ability of their staff the Diner never missed a beat.

This period in Traveler's life was probably his biggest spiritual shift. He became a student of self-development and read as many self-help and spiritual books as he could lay his hands on. The under-lying message was always the same in all success stories as they attributed their accomplishments only to their Source. Life stories & situations that seemed insurmountable for one person but through an attitude of never giving up they reached their goals. Traveler began to see God as being much closer in his life not as some Entity in Heaven but a source of one's power within. Traveler was already a relatively quiet person and rarely became angry but now there was a little more peace inside. He was still determined to eliminate that little doll called stress out of his life along with her luggage. When he became strong enough to venture from the house, he began making trips to the local Book Store to find the next piece of this puzzle called Truth. He became intent on finding the Truth in all areas of his life and how it related to existence here on Earth.

One of the books he had bought was on learning how to meditate. He had had it at home for a while but its' funny how one gets programmed to fear the unknown, so he was hesitant to give it a try. One evening he was staying alone at home and decided that today was the day. He made himself comfortable sitting on the bedroom floor and began as per the instructions in this little book. He was trying to keep his upper body straight while quieting the mind, a far bigger challenge than he had ever imagined. The body ached, whined and was adamant about wanting to lie down, all this while the mind rifled in thought after thought without end. Traveler was determined to get beyond this and began focusing his breath on a point at the end of his nose, just like the book indicated, in and out until that point began to hurt. Finally, the mind became quiet, and the body started to straighten on its' own, taking the weighted feeling away from him. His arms began to slide off his lap which kind of alarmed him, but he was mentally ready for any experience. They slide onto the floor and then continued upwards until they were perfectly touching palm to palm above his head almost pulling him up. Within a few moments he had lost all sense of his body and his presence remained in or as a bright light with the only sound that existed was that of the blood rushing through his heart in a steady beat. The perfect peacefulness, a place where he wanted to remain, then a thought, of how could he ever share this experience, who would believe him. Traveler considered that night as a gift, he knew without a doubt that our presence here on Earth was more than the body and mind. He was once again filled with optimism and renewed energy for this journey which many times has us traveling by our self (little ego) but over time the journey is spent more in awareness with your Self. Integration with your Thought Adjuster, that Divine connection to Source, takes time and much effort.

Traveler returned to work once again at the Diner after about four months, but he was far from healed and even though he had returned to this fast pace, he did not have the strength. It was now coming up to the five-year date that they had originally set when stepping into the Restaurant business and he knew without a doubt that it was time to step out of it. Fran was well rooted in their Diner life and enjoyed working with the staff and had become good friends with many of their customers, but this young Traveler was burnt out.

Syl was becoming a little disillusioned with the Amway business by this time and during the following few months he made the decision to purchase the Diner. By June of 1995 Traveler was now able to sit at the counter of this little Diner as a customer. It was an emotional time for their family and the staff as they had become close, sharing each other's life. There were not many changes in the Restaurant during those five years but the changes within Traveler were profound.

CREATOR'S HAND

Looking back Traveler could not believe how strong the ego and mind are. They had sold the Diner so he could rest and take a little time to gather his thoughts but within three weeks he was traveling to Quebec for a meeting with a Franchisor to discuss the purchase of another ongoing business in the city. The ego needs attachment, it needs to feel important and distinctive, and it does not care whether it is poor health or success as long as it has something to cling to. The ego and its' desire to be busy prevailed and within a month or so they now owned a bottled water distributor license agreement for their area.

There is no doubt that the Universe continues to present so many wonderful opportunities in our lives, but it is here where discernment is necessary. Yes, action is required but it is better not to chase it, listen to your heart and ask through your inner connection, "Is this right for me?" and wait for an answer. It might take a day or a week, but if you have confidence in Source, the answer will come and you will be sure that it is in alignment with the Divine Idea, not just a thought in your mind.

This is a point in the story where all hell began to break loose within the family unit. Rory had been progressing along fairly well, having a normal teenager's life with sports and studies in High School taking up the better part of his time. Charlotte had spent the summer working at the horse stable, riding her horse and then at the end of Summer, started her first year of High School. She had been an above average student in Elementary School so common sense would say that that would continue. This fork in the road was not really Traveler's but the ripple effect from Charlotte's decisions was life changing for sure.

Fran and Traveler had a little different philosophy on raising children as she preferred to be a little strict while he liked to give Rory and Charlotte room to grow as an adult, more freedom, and a chance to adventure, like he had done in his youth. Somewhere in between might have brought more balance into the family, but no one knows the Divine plan. Traveler was not sure whether a parent could guide a child's life as they are here, as most souls, part of a higher plan to explore and experience. If the parents give their unconditional love, provide a safe home environment, a place where they can rest and experience family, then outside of that should be some freedom for the adventure. Children are wonderful teachers; they can help us grow if we are attentive, in ways unimaginable.

Charlotte seemed to begin her school year as most students do and be progressing along normally. She had some exceptionally good friends, but she also had a few that were helping her go left at the fork in the road or maybe it was a joint effort. Traveler had learned early on not to condemn the efforts of parents on how they raised their children as it was clearly a challenge, and attaining perfection, was a near impossible dream. He was trying to pull the reins in a little on their horseback rider, going over the list of respect, attitude etc. but Charlotte was keeping the reins tight and swinging for freedom.

The reality of her daily adventure hit home when the Hospital called to say that Charlotte was brought into emergency after smoking some bad weed at school. Those calls can be a little scary and humbling especially if the parents are not aware of the smoking habit. Fran was going through a stressful time at work with cutbacks in the Health Care System that were having a dramatic effect on all staff members, and she really was not prepared physically or emotionally to handle Charlotte's attitude on life. Traveler's uncle shared one day the words of his Father, simply said "We look after our own."

The hallway in their home became an emotional sparring ground for Fran and Charlotte, sharp words and neither one giving an inch. Fathers are usually accused or perhaps are guilty of having a soft spot for their daughters, but Traveler felt an equal love for both his children. This love has the same depth, but the relationship is different as with any other being. He soon became the referee, not an enviable position and he mentally hit the mat a few times wishing for a quiet space, as was Fran. Traveler was being driven deeper within, looking for some peace, some happiness, and ultimately the Truth.

About the same time, Rory had made it to the hospital a couple times for stiches etc. He had flown off the front of his friend's Van, and yes, alcohol was involved this time and with a few other accidents, but the bright side was that they always made it home.

The following Summer after Charlotte completed her first year of high school a mutual decision was made among Traveler, Fran and Charlotte, that she would attend a private school which was located almost an hour from their home. After many months with their nerves on edge, it appeared to be the solution. There were a few reasons for choosing this school. It had a strict dress code helping to eliminate peer pressure, it also had fewer students per Teacher allowing for more individual attention with each student and it was far enough away to help severe the ties of influence from a few of her friends. Another fork in the road, let us see what happens.

It had taken most of their reserve cash and more to make this opportunity come into reality for Charlotte, but it was a non-issue. Traveler had had little time to devote to their water business and this upcoming year would not change that. Charlotte was off to a rocky start that Autumn, trying to fit in and testing the severity of the school's disciplinary action. Traveler was beginning to wear a path making the trips back and forth to the school trying to keep her focused on remaining there.

It was on a Sunday where Charlotte and Traveler had spent part of the day together touring the countryside and small towns near the school, and it was time for her to return for the evening. They walked up the stairs through the front door and went into the sitting room next to the reception area and front desk. Charlotte looked at Traveler with her dark brown eyes wanting to make sure that she had his attention. She reiterated on how strict the school was and how determined she was to return home to finish her high school year. It was not a new discussion, but this moment was brimming with a room full of emotion. Charlotte threatened to run away from school if she could not return home. With all the strength left in Traveler's heart, he said to her that if she chose to leave the school and walked down the driveway to the open gate, she should turn right, away from home because she couldn't return there until the school year was completed. He told Charlotte that he loved her unconditionally, the decision was hers and he turned to walk away. With the two ladies at the reception area tuned into every word of this conversation Charlotte yelled out, "What kind of father would leave his daughter in a hell hole like this?" He felt weak at the knees as he walked down the front steps but managed to return to his car. On the trip home Traveler felt sick going over in his mind whether his decision to be tough was the right one.

Charlotte phoned the next day to apologize and to say that she was ready to stick it out and complete her year.

It was an unbearable time for Fran with nowhere to run or hide as hospital cutbacks made for an unpleasant workplace and home didn't feel much like home. The phone ringing became more like a fire alarm and chances were that it was the Dean of the school giving them a report on Charlotte's day.

Charlotte had become quite familiar with the campus chapel not only from participating in the service but also from cleaning it so often. Cleaning the chapel was part of the school's disciplinary action for misbehaving students. Thank God that the school did not give up and neither did Fran or Traveler, as each week seemed to present a challenge, but they stayed the course.

Often in our life it seems like there are events that help us connect the dots and change our path. We are all connected by a fine thread as people come into our life to offer information that can help improve the quality of our experience. During that year, the nurse at school felt that maybe some of Charlotte's behavior was being caused by A.D.D., although it was becoming a popular term used for children that were having difficulty concentrating Traveler did not agree with her suggestion. Creator's presence is usually very subtle but undeniable our lives.

Traveler was at the local gym one morning and picked up a magazine getting ready for a bike ride. It was not long after he started pedaling that he found a smaller magazine stuck to the one that he had picked up. The complete front cover was referring to an article on Attention Deficit Disorder written by Maggie who was involved in a Naturopathic Clinic in Toronto. He finally reached out to Maggie by phone later that same day and within their conversation she began to enlighten Traveler on health issues.

Maggie had beaten terminal cancer about ten years prior mainly through self-discipline, determination, and ongoing research on alternative healing. Traveler explained Charlotte's situation, but it wasn't long into their conversation that she was asking about Traveler's life history. He soon began to realize that his farming days had given him more than just memories. As he continued to give a detail of his life to date; Maggie asked how his mental state was and he knew exactly what she meant. His health had been on a downhill slide for several years but after having pneumonia it was picking up the pace. He would eat lunch and within twenty minutes he felt like his body had been run over by a truck and many times he would have to lay down for half an hour to get over it. Doctor's comments were usually to the affect that it was all in his mind or just stress, hence the reason for Maggie's question. Traveler's response to Maggie was that his mental state was good mainly because he had been buried in self-help and spiritual study for a few years. She said that he was fortunate as many people ended up with mental problems because they began to believe that all their physical illnesses were in their mind.

Although chemicals were being used commercially after the end of WWII, the home farm did not start using them until the mid-1960s. There were no warnings on the dangers of DDT or Atrazine to one's health, so it was just a matter of getting the right mix in the tank and begin spraying. If the wind was blowing it into their face, it was an inconvenience, but they never really gave serious thought to the damage it might cause to their health. Traveler had had his foot caught in a corn auger when he was seventeen which opened up a wound where mold and bacteria could enter. In fact, he was breathing toxic mold in every time the corn needed to be shoveled around in the storage bin. He started wearing a dust mask in the barn when he was twenty-five because he was having a hard time breathing with the dust especially during feeding. The list that he was giving Maggie was endless as they put the pieces of the puzzle together.

Maggie began to explain the effects of Candida, a bacteria that makes up part of the flora in everyone but when given an opportunity it can become overpopulated and a detriment to the health of the body and eventually the mind, both physically and emotionally. It can migrate to any part of the body and flourish to a point where the immune system will not challenge it anymore. Traveler had fog in his head since High School and a ringing in his ears that blocked out all other sound sometimes, but one can become accustomed to these quirks thinking that it is normal. Maggie said that it was probable that Charlotte and even Rory may be feeling the effects of an overgrowth of Candida. Antibiotics which were often given to their children for sore throats or ear infection can kill most of the flora in our digestive system and if not rebuilt with fresh organic yogurt or living acidophilus, an imbalance can quickly occur. Maggie had turned the light on and opened a door to an understanding of this new world of well-being. An appointment was set for Charlotte and Traveler and within ten days they were sitting in Maggie's office.

Traveler was excited but with reservation as alternative medicine was something new for him. Uncle Allan had normally looked after any major illnesses in the family. That is where the confusion can lie; curing a sickness with antibiotics can work but healing requires an effort of bringing the body/mind back to a healthy state of origin. Maggie went into a bit of her own personal history and then talked with Traveler alone and then Charlotte later that morning.

Maggie introduced them to her partner Helena a Naturopathic Doctor at the clinic. Helena completed tests and blood work on both Charlotte and Traveler and within a week they both returned for an analysis of the results. Although some of the mineral and blood analyses took another two weeks to complete, they had enough information to get started. It was confirmed that both Charlotte and Traveler had exceptionally high levels of Candida. His level was about ten to eleven times higher than normal resulting in the body rejecting most of his diet. Each time he ate something, the food appeared as an antigen signaling an attack from the immune system. Maggie had given him a couple of books to help educate himself on the effects of food on a human's health. By mid-day they were ready to head back home, with their homeopathic drops etc., vitamins and renewed hope on this path to health. They were given an antibiotic to knock the Candida and a guideline for a change of diet, to limit the regrowth of this bacteria. Back at school they were informed of the health treatment that Charlotte was on and with the help of the school nurse and the kitchen staff it was implemented.

The diet that was required to try and eliminate this imbalance in his body, seemed almost impossible but Traveler was determined and after one week on the program he could not believe the change in how he felt. His mind was clearing, and the body was slowly lifting its' weighted feeling. He was hooked and thought, if this program can make such a dramatic change in his life in one week how much different would the level of his health be in one year. He quickly found out that almost every product in the grocery store aisles contain processed wheat or sugar (even sugar in table salt) and more often than not, both ingredients. Health food stores in the early 1990s were almost non- existent in their area and soon his search brought him to Ottawa and there he thought that he was in Heaven with the selection of food available to fit his new diet.

They traveled to Toronto every three to four weeks to check on their progress and make any necessary adjustments. Traveler had shed quite a few pounds and was now down to a level that he had not seen since about grade 11 in High School. Relatives & friends concluded that he was severely ill because of the weight loss and the regular trips to this so-called clinic. A change in perception does not come easy for most, still stuck in an old program. Traveler continued to follow the protocol precisely and with each passing week his well-being continued to improve. Through this experience his family became aware of the effect that food can have on your health. For many years after, he became a student of this information determined to fine tune his health which continued to improve year after year.

Creator had been instrumental in many changes in his life whether he was conscious or not. This awareness, brought to light through Maggie and Helena's knowledge, helped to put the pieces of the puzzle together to continue finding a way to inner peace. It allowed him an opportunity to experience his Inner-Self without limitations caused from poor health. If the mind is only focused on the poor health of the body, then there is little chance of stopping those thoughts to be at peace. There would be new challenges arising but one step at a time.

During this time Traveler's efforts in the Amway business had slowed considerably although he was still consuming a constant feed of tapes and books through their organization along with any other spiritual information he could find. Fran came home from work one day and said that they were invited to meet with a couple from Ottawa and listen to a business opportunity that they were presenting. It was being arranged through one of Fran's co-workers and so off they went. Another fork in the road, another experience waiting to unfold.

NETWORK MARKETING RETURNS

Neil and Jeannette were a dynamic couple full of energy and as Fran & Traveler soon found out, truly knowledgeable in network marketing. Neil had built a successful Amway business which was still producing a residual income month after month, but during much of his career he had also been studying the cycle of industries. He had been searching since the mid-1980s for a company that would lead the industry in break through the barriers of non-acceptance with the general public. Neil felt that he had found the company with the right compensation plan and upper management. Neil was nearing the completion of a thirty-five-year long career with the Federal Government but his and Jeannette's enthusiasm for the network marketing industry was contagious. Fran and Traveler made a mutual decision to become part of Neil & Jeannette's business and the fact that the product was Jewelry had Fran excited about participating.

They had just sold their Water Distributorship, so they decided to build this network marketing business full time. With Fran's enthusiasm for the product and their desire for financial freedom they developed a large organization of people within a few months. It was a great time as they met many wonderful people who through this business shared some of their own life challenges. One Lady who Traveler always held in high esteem was Rita. She had decided late in life to change career paths and without looking back became one of the most successful Financial Planners in her area. There were many other Ladies that he looked up to with respect for their determination and successes in life.

They became good friends with Neil & Jeannette and there was hardly a week went by that they were not together holding a meeting or training sessions. Joey had jumped on board once again and they soon found themselves on the plane heading to Tucson for the company's annual convention. This company had had significant growth and was now expanding into Europe. They were already number three in North American sales and their future looked bright. Only one slight problem was that it appeared that government was not totally on board with the network marketing industry yet and still looking for ways to stagger its' growth. Within less than a year the government had successfully shut the company down. Interestingly enough the founder was a chartered accountant and managed the company's daily operations with the utmost care. It was disappointing but there are many things in life that we are not able to change, so we move on. It was a moment for reflection, where can a person place trust in the outside world.

It was another fork in the road moment for Traveler, but change was a part of his life, for many others who saw their income drop to zero and a complete loss of livelihood in some cases, it was devastating.

Traveler liked to say that he stopped there but he had developed a fondness for the industry and for sales. Being involved in the industry had broadened his scope and understanding of the world, at least a little. Many of the books that he had read on success stories were about people who were in sales where there were no limitations other than their own.

He continued the journey with self-development being one of his main focuses. Every situation in life has possibilities, good and not so good. It was through the jewelry business that Traveler had had the pleasure of meeting Gerry the owner of a Dale Carnegie franchise in Ottawa. Joey and he signed up for the course and started the weekly drive to the capital city to try and overcome the fear of public speaking. Yes, the little self-doubt demon was still with him after all these years.

It was an evening course and when they first started class there were about 30 people and within a couple of weeks the group was down to about 20 participants. Traveler looked at all of these people and wandered where the fear was as most of them looked fairly comfortable giving their three-minute talks in class. Many of them were executives working for different companies including one Lady who often sat beside him. She was thinking of quitting because she could not handle the fear, after Traveler explained his own hurdles, she figured she could tough it out and stayed to complete her course.

There were always two chairs set up at the back of the room where you would go and sit when you thought you were ready to get up in front of the group and speak. If you waited too long, then the fear would just build, so usually Joey and Traveler were back there quickly. Johnny humor was with Traveler once again trying to take people's attention away from him while the instructor tried to keep him on track. Their group became quite close as they begin to share stories about their personal life usually saved for close friends or family. Traveler began to see the underlying pain that most people carried throughout their lives but like him, they had kept it buried as a possible fault or flaw, not able to see its origin. Many of their memories which were now the cause of this pain, feeling of shame or self-doubt were covered layer after layer making this impediment more difficult to heal. This mask that people consciously or unconsciously put on before they head out the door in the morning to face the day is normally not the original. There is the potential of three characters in one, the one that this person thinks he is, appearance in all aspects of his life. Then there is the one that other people perceive as they scan features, characteristics and quickly without further study decide who that person is. In rare occasions there is that person who is comfortable with who they are and actually love themselves, demonstrating in confidence, the original.

This somewhat renowned Dale Carnegie course was a success for Traveler as it helped to remove a lot of that inner fear that had been with him most of his life. Perhaps he was not ready to speak in front of hundreds quite yet but at least the thought of it did not make him feel sick anymore. Evolution seems like a slow process for humanity, taking thousands and thousands of years, or quite possibly thousands of lifetimes to make a shift from the caveman's state of survival and depending on the situation, fight, or flight. It will take some assistance from our cosmic brothers and sisters but perhaps not so far in our future we will see a conscious shift to unity, harmonization of all lifeforms here on earth, working together towards a better world. Each human experience brings with it an opportunity to integrate with that Divine Presence within, yet so many lifetimes are spent fully engaged to the outside world. There is nothing wrong with being part of the world, that is why we are here, but we are supposed to be awake. All souls have the opportunity while experiencing life as human beings to continue move freely in spirit to other time spaces. All of our growth as a soul takes effort to find our unique path homeward where we begin to spend more time in spirit. As we begin to live more in spirit, we gain abilities that help us to truly see another being going beyond their physical characteristics and even beyond their emotional state to see that spark of life within them, to see beyond the mask.

By the time the school year was over in 1997, the family had purchased a home near Martintown and once again they were back to country living. This home was situated on three acres of land which included a small, wooded area and a spring fed pond. Rory was still continually active in hockey, so the vision of a large skating rink on the pond came to mind and then a reality. They were quite familiar with this home as it sat across from their original family farm and also close to Sam and Penny's log home. This brick house had been built by the MacCallums circa 1847. They were an affluent family during the early settlement of the village and contributed to the growth of the community.

They were all anxious to be a part of this country community again and enjoy the peacefulness that it offers. It was an opportunity for Charlotte to complete her school studies closer to home, where her parents had enjoyed their high school years. Sam and Penny were now well into their retirement years and were excited about having more family close at hand, along with Jim's family who lived just down the road on another farm. The property required some tender loving care, but they could see the potential and were ready to begin the transformation.

Traveler's office was set up in the sun porch on the upper level of their home, overlooking the previous family farm. Perhaps it was God's sense of humor but also it was an opportunity to further develop non-attachment to this physical world and the material objects within it.

They had received a beautiful leather-bound Bible from John and Ruth on their wedding day and Traveler thought perhaps now after twenty years it would be the time to study its' teachings. He had tried reading the Bible off and on during his life and this time was not much different as he could not comprehend the old text, so he continued his study through other people's writing and experiences.

They soon had the property cleaned up, green grass growing and ready for a fresh cut. There were many huge maple trees that dotted the property line and a few fruit trees behind the house. It was so peaceful and blissful to live there and be close to the family. Traveler's parents enjoyed watching the changes on the property and father Sam was always anxious to lend a hand and his equipment. Slowly the vision began to unfold in their minds as plans were made for a post and beam structure to replace the building which now held a hot tub and pool, which were no longer in use.

It was during this time that Traveler began using the power of thought and spending as much time as possible building the vision of this property in his mind while living in gratitude for all that they had in their lives. The exercise is most difficult, not so much in the forming of the vision but to bring the mind back to that creative faculty, as the ego prefers to keep it active on other daily activities and thoughts. It is most important to keep all disruptive and negative thoughts away from the mind. He used to imagine that his mind was a beautiful, enclosed garden with sliding doors to enter or leave. If there were any negative thoughts or feelings, he would sweep them out beyond the doors and then quickly close them. It became a highly effective way to keep his mind centered and maintain the vision. You can be compassionate about the pain and suffering of others but do not absorb that energy. At first glance, it may seem that you lack compassion but as the Wingmakers say in a song, "the other side of compassion." it requires an understanding. Later in Traveler's life this understanding of creating would change, but for now in the physical/material world it was effective.

Winter had settled in and on a dark January night in 1998 most of Eastern Ontario was about to experience the worst natural disaster that it had ever seen. Freezing rain is a common occurrence especially in January but normally it changes to rain or snow with little damage resulting, just slippery roads and walkways. This storm was different as it continued throughout the next day and by the following evening the damage was almost terrifying. As they lay in bed trying to sleep the sounds of branches cracking and then hitting the ground was heart wrenching. When daylight came, their property looked like the loggers had been working all night as limbs and branches covered the lawn. There was no time for grieving as the community was soon without electricity. News traveled around the area as to the extent of the damage. Hydro poles were being knocked down like toothpicks and even many of the steel towers were buckling under the weight of the ice. Any of the trees that did not break were bent over to caress the ground and remain there until spring and beyond.

The first couple of days passed by with candlelight dinners served hot off the barbeque. Sam and Penny would brave the slippery trek over to Traveler's place to dine. This was fun for the first week but soon the novelty wore off and the reality had set in. Before long members of our Army arrived to help those in need. Generators were coming in from all areas of the province to help farmers continue to milk cows and feed livestock. Jim was floating a generator from house to house to give everybody a fresh supply of water each day and run the furnace for a while to take the chill out of their homes. They were fortunate because they had wood fireplaces to keep the frost from freezing the water pipes, well most of them at least. Sequins from up the road were like elves bringing firewood to those without which included Traveler's family.

As devastating as the situation was it brought the village and surrounding area closer together to share the hardship. Martintown's Community Center became the mess hall as people brought in food from their freezers and families shared time together cooking meals to serve all that stopped by. It was a God sent for many of the elderly in the area that did not have the means to look after themselves. It was three weeks before Traveler had power restored to his home and for many in outlying areas it was well over a month. Spring was a time for a cleanup of the damage and soon the Ice Storm of 1998 was just a memory written into history.

Nature has quite a force and when her balance is disrupted, she can sure devastate an area in a hurry. There are many factors that are affecting Mother Earth and have been for a long, long time. Blue skies were the norm here on the planet, clouds rolling in when moisture was needed all existing in harmony. Today chem trails, dark clouds that float by with no intention of rain and many other alterations in our climate, are the effects of humans interfering with nature, rarely does that have beneficial long-term results. Human experience, for much of the population, is lived under the harmful grid of electrical and telecommunication lines. Traveler remembers the negative affect these lines had on dairy herds, dropping their milk production, affecting their general health and many times causing death. Humans have been numbed down for so long that they do not notice what is going on around them anymore, dreaming during the night and sleeping during the day. The Truth is always present, we just have to start looking…

It had been a long, difficult Winter and a bit of a strain which was affecting the harmony in Traveler's family, so the decision was made to purchase a pup. They are animals that share their love freely and are well known for their healing capabilities. They had been searching for a Basenji for almost three years and had finally found a breeder in the State of Pennsylvania who had a litter of pups. Charlotte and Traveler made the trip to Pennsylvania early one morning and spent a few hours with the family and a home full of little Basenji's. Breeders are quick to interview you and want to know your knowledge on the breed as they are not for everyone. Traveler was quite fond of the Basenji breed since the family had had one on the farm when he was 12 years old. Meru was brought over from Africa by a local Doctor but after a few months of this beautiful pet being confined to a home in the city, they realized that Meru needed more space to burn off his energy. They are one of the most intelligent animals on earth and in play they can usually out smart most humans, yes even Traveler.

One of the larger males in the litter seem to pick Charlotte and Traveler as companions and by late afternoon they were heading North with Johnnie. It was not the normal African name that usually befits a Basenji but there was a little humor behind picking the name and so it remained. Johnnie stayed true and lived up to his ability to love and be loved although there are many that would not agree as he was always cautious about making new friends quickly. Johnnie soon had harmony back in their home and a new beginning with the arrival of Spring.

During the past couple of years Traveler and Fran had kept in contact with Neil and Jeannette. One day they called Traveler charged with an excitement that had reached a new high after returning from a Financial Seminar in the Bahamas. After a few months of gentle persuasion Fran and Traveler along with a few other friends were on a flight to Aruba to attend the June seminar. Although Jeannette had described briefly what the format was at the conference none of the group were prepared for the information that was delivered by different speakers during that week.

They would all meet for an evening meal after the day's sessions and review all that had been presented by the speakers. The information was a bit overwhelming, and Traveler wandered how he could have been so naïve about life, but each day brought with it a feeling of freedom just in knowing some of the truth about the world they were living in. There was a broad spectrum of topics some of which included the education system, banking industry, health care and many controlling factors that influenced governments and hence most countries throughout the world. "The Creature from Jekyll Island" written by Edward Griffin, would be a great start to get an overall sense of how a few people take advantage of the world's population, mostly for their benefit and agenda. Traveler returned home after that week with a whole new outlook on life and wanting to share it with the world. If one starts to look for Truth it will eventually begin to flow towards you, one just needs to be open to receive.

With renewed enthusiasm the vision for renovations to their country home continued to build in Traveler's mind. The property was now starting to take shape as was the picture in his mind, constantly trying to keep the vision at the fore front, leaning towards it. All souls are co-creators some consciously, many not… Every thought has power, and every word, even more. Father Sam often repeated this mantra, "If you have nothing good to say about another, best not to say anything." If we began there, it would be a great start to becoming less judgmental concerning another of our fellow human beings.

By September Joey and Traveler were on a flight to Mexico to meet brother Hugh and attend the Fall seminar. Hugh had lived a string of successes in his life and was much more conservative in his thinking than Traveler, but he was willing to expand his perception of the world, especially the part on taxation. After the completion of the first day of the Seminar, everyone shared the same sentiments once again, how could they have been kept in the dark about this information all their lives. There was no doubt that the information was somewhat liberating, but it was almost beyond many people's concept of how they could be so blind. A banking system that created money out of thin air, central banks controlled by private corporations, yes even Canada's. It was like an open door to another world, and many stepped through with caution and carefully looked around, a few made the choice to look no further and return to their habitual life. That was not Traveler's nature, and he was well beyond the door searching behind every tree for more truth, more freedom. There had been segments during that week's talk on the world's different religions and at the forefront was the catholic churches and their wide swath of control over governments. There is a lot of truth bearing information on all of these topics and there is also much of it that is badly distorted, this is where your own discernment comes into play.

There are many scandals about priests throughout many countries, Canada is no exception and there were quite a few incidents in and around Traveler's home area. On the brighter side, many of the local priests turned to alcohol on a regular basis, perhaps to numb the facts about their brotherhood but more likely just a way of enjoyment or a time to reflect on their life choices. As was the norm for a few years, Traveler would accompany his parents for Sunday mass. The priest was a local boy and knew father Sam quite well. It was a ritual each Sunday for the three of them to sit on the back pew where father Sam could be found quickly slipping towards a nap which was usually long before mass started. Father Calvin would make his trip down the center aisle to greet everyone on the way and eventually pass by the bowl of holy water where he would dip one hand in. Like clockwork every Sunday he would flick the water on the back of Sam's neck and startle him out of his sleep. They were both predictable, but they always laughed.

One other Sunday morning the three of them attending the same mass only with a different priest. It was an early mass, so the church was not too full. All was quiet, waiting for the priest to enter and begin, but after ten minutes or so, there was still no sign of him. Finally, a couple of directors of the church went to find Father G… They came back with him one on each side guiding their priest along as he was still entrenched in the effects of alcohol from the night before. The boys finally got him up front and leaned him onto the pulpit. He slurred out a short version of "Our Father Who Art in Heaven", blessed himself and the directors quickly helped him back to the Rectory. It was for sure the shortest service that anyone had ever experienced.

It takes a while to wrap the mind around the idea of oneness or even unity, not too sure that the human mind can fully perceive it. There are so many memories to let go of, before a human being can begin to understand this unity of consciousness. This body that one is born into, already has memories from previous life experiences that need to be addressed or cleared, but it is enough just to begin releasing experiences from this lifetime. It is not so easy when one is not awake yet. Understanding is one key but how does a person reach a higher understanding, keep reaching for the Truth, although ever changing, it is not so far away. You must ask for guidance from within and start to develop trust in this Source and continue with your search through books that you are drawn to. Many times, you will read something that confirms exactly what you saw in a vision or in meditation.

For the following three years Traveler never missed a seminar. He began to bring other people, who were at least interested in becoming aware of this information and perhaps change their perception of life and their experience within it. Within a short period of time, Traveler began working for one of the Presenters at these events. It was a wonderful moment in his life combining travel with friends and associates while gaining a better understanding with each trip. He was meeting many people from different countries who were of the same mindset and the energy seemed magical, quite liberating.

All that Traveler had studied for many years and put into daily practice started to change his reality. His faith or trust in Creator deepened as did his gratitude for all that was flowing into his life. One beautiful warm Summer afternoon gave Traveler a chance to see the fragility of life. His daughter came up to the office to say that she was going out with her friends, gave her dad a kiss and headed out the door. Charlotte had her own car by then and was only about five kilometers from home when she lost control of the vehicle. It flipped side to side and end to end before it came crashing down beside a hydro pole. Just a couple of minutes after Charlotte had pulled out of the driveway, Traveler closed the computer and called it a day. He walked into his bedroom, dropped to his knees giving gratitude to God for all that had come into his family's life, for this moment of bliss and asked for protection for Charlotte and Rory during the night. It was about ten minutes later when the phone rang, it was Charlotte calling to say that she had been in an accident but was she was okay…

By the beginning of 2001 they had plans in place to begin construction that Spring for the post & beam addition to their home. One should be aware of what they wish for and how powerful it can become when written on paper. Fran and Traveler had always talked about living on a farm East of the Village. It had a beautiful two-hundred-year-old stone home sitting on a hill a good distance from the road and overlooked a mile of farmland to the south. They had kind of put it out of their mind thinking that it would not come up for sale. Their family had farmed the land for a number of years, so they were quite familiar with the property.

In 1995 Traveler had written a date and a list of things as part of his goals and vision. It was for this farm to become their home and the construction of an addition and restoration that would be completed in the fall of 2001. At that moment in 1995, it was beyond comprehension how it would become a reality because at that time, there was little equity left in their home and savings were non-existent. This farm came up for sale early in the Spring of 2001, a month or so before they were to start renovations on their home. Uncle Allan, stopped by one day while out for a drive and said, "I suppose you'll be buying the farm". "What farm?" was Traveler's response. Uncle Al said, "The one that you've always wanted". Traveler did not know that it had come up for sale, but now the seed was planted. Yes, thought is powerful and by the end of that year, after a Summer of construction, clearing trees, picking stones and planting grass, they had moved into a dream that had started 20 years prior and put into a clear vision 6 years before the move.

It is hard to describe the beauty that this property has, at least with Traveler's perception of it. Waking up each morning felt like they were in a country resort and the feeling was the same day after day. The farm was a place where the dogs could run free, which seemed to fill Fran's heart with bliss. Fran always had a magic touch for decorating and this home was a place for her to express herself and bring it to its' full potential. When Traveler tired of the phone he would step out the porch door and continue with the never-ending landscaping work that the property had to offer. He was attached to every aspect of this dream.

He had met many wonderful people through his travels and during one of the seminars he had an opportunity to meet Harv Ecker. Harv's company called Peak Potentials was helping people break free of their habitual nature and realize their full potential. Within a couple of months Rory and Traveler were on a flight to Calgary and then onward to Red Deer to spend a weekend at a Peak Potential Seminar. Traveler felt that this information would be helpful to Charlotte and Rory to start out their adult life and by the end of the weekend the three of them were scheduled in for August to participate in Harv's Enlightened Warrior Camp in the foothills of the Rockies.

Charlotte came by bus to Calgary from Whistler where she was living at the time and Rory flew in from Toronto where he was working. The three of them headed North, full of anticipation for the upcoming week. Traveler will respect Harv's wishes and not share the events of that week, but it was life changing for all of them. During their five night stay they did not sleep much more than 20 hours, as facilitators worked their magic slowly transforming the group. Harv repeated many times when the body is tired the mind becomes open to change. Yoga which started at 6:30 in the morning was a life saver as it rejuvenated everyone's weary bodies. Yoga became a practice that the three of them continue today. Early Friday morning they were packed and heading to their separate homes with an event routed deep in their hearts where it remains vivid today. Rory and Charlotte were able to attend Harv's Wizard Camp, two years later which took them to a new level of experience and understanding in spirituality. Rory had an experience one evening where he was consciously aware of each person talking and what was being said within this group of 100 people. It was a shift for him and as well for Charlotte.

Traveler has a strong belief in being focused on two aspects of life, one being Spirit, in connection to our human experience and the other being health, they are inter-related. One cannot experience either one fully without the other. There have been many Healers that came into his life including Chiropractors, Naturopaths, Homeopaths, Kinesiology Practitioners, and Massage Therapists. Without a doubt one of the most beneficial, was Wen Shu an Acupuncturist who was able to remove many deep-seated energy blockages. An emotional or physical trauma can be the beginning of deep-seated pain or even illness. One example is when Traveler had a hernia at age fourteen and was operated on to repair the tear in his lower abdomen. There was a fair bit of trauma before going into the operating room as the drug was causing nausea and along with this came a feeling of anxiety until finally the anesthesia put him to sleep. This operation was successful but as the years went on the scar tissue became extremely sensitive to touch. It was through the Acupuncturist that the healing took place. It took quite a supply of acupuncture needles each week along with grueling massage that many times caused so much discomfort that Traveler wanted to cry. The healing should have been done right after the operation, to release all these energies of pain, anxiety, and fear to name a few, but who would have known that. During thirty-five years of Traveler's life this area of discomfort was holding other moments or memories of pain, anxiety, and fear. It became a collection point of deep-rooted memories, blocked until one day they could finally be released. When pain and sickness come up to the surface, it is the body's way of saying, liberate them. The treatment could not be effective with one or two tries, each time the pain was located deeper within that area, so it was necessary to massage the area deeper until the pain was liberated. It is a step-by-step process or treatment as the Practitioner cannot get to the original memory on the first try, it is like releasing the memories one by one. There are many ways to clear these memories. Someone who has experience in energy work can bring enough light in to clear the memory but again there may be more than one. It is much more beneficial if the patient closes his eyes and permits the memories of these incidents to come to mind. Once the memory is clear and you can see or remember it, go back to that moment, feel that the pain or emotion is real, and then give support and love to yourself, such as holding yourself as a child until all that negative energy or memory has dissipated. Forgive any others who were there at that moment and give them love for their misperception or lack of understanding. There are many good Healers on earth at this time that can help with this process. This is just scratching the surface of what work is required to clean up the memories of the body and mind, but each moment of release or healing is liberating, slowly bringing one back to a peaceful state of being.

A REAL FORK IN THE ROAD

During and after Enlightened Warrior Camp, Traveler had experienced a feeling of love for all his fellow humans, a feeling of being a part of them and although it was difficult to sustain as he was being slowly pulled back into the so-called real world, it continued resonating in his heart. It faded over the following few weeks, but memory of that feeling was an unmistakable shift in his outlook on life. He decided that somehow, he wanted to reach that level of awareness again through meditation and diet. He began to meditate each morning at 5:00 o'clock and decided to try and eliminate alcohol from his life. There were intervals during his life where he had quit drinking but each time it was difficult to stay the course as socially the friends and family have a difficult time accepting it. What do you mean you quit drinking and "Where's the sense in that?" here get that into you… It would be easier for Traveler to stay at home, but they all came for a visit anyway. This time lasted almost a year with the exception of a glass of wine now and then. Meditation for Traveler became an addiction as each blissful experience seated a strong desire for the next experience, similar to alcohol but without the hangover and a feeling of helplessness for a few days. Anyone who drinks alcohol excessively knows the routine. Although part of the illusion, it seems that the only way out lies in the next round of beer and booze. It is a fact that an excessive consumption of alcohol can slowly drain your life away and many times the life of others close to you. There is no right or wrong in these life choices, just depends on how a soul wants to journey through the experience. These extreme ways of living are like the movement of a pendulum, they can eventually bring you back to your center or balance.

For almost a year most of his time was spent working on their farm property, trying to bring it back to its original beauty, that which had been hidden with an overgrowth of vines and poor-quality trees. He would step away from the office as often as possible to continue with this passion of being a part of the dream unfolding. Traveler can safely say that he could have spent the remainder of his days participating in this labor of love.

Fran and Traveler had had many family gatherings on the farm, and they were always anxious to share its peacefulness and beauty with others. As a couple they had had some rough periods in their time together and especially so over the past ten years. They had become calm, more peaceful inside, but they had grown apart or at least Traveler had.

Their life was near perfect except for that one underlying feeling that he couldn't mask. Each day he was willing to go beyond it and just enjoy all that they had been blessed with in their lives but eventually it became a source of discomfort for both of them.

There are plans in place for the experience (or the unfoldment of it) as our soul is born into this human instrument in order to fully engage with the emotional and physical capabilities of this body. It is not an easy adventure here on earth but one that many souls want to experience. One could go against the grain but if not in this life than in another the soul lives out the adventure that is part of Creator's desire to explore Its creation. Traveler was never much in tune with Astrology or the movements of our planets and Sun, but he became more aware of the significance of their alignments. In the Fall of 2003 Venus was at its closest point to Earth and it was incredible to watch its brightness from the farm. One evening the planet was so bright it seemed to be glowing in through their bedroom windows. It was about 3:00 o'clock in the morning Traveler woke up and decided to go outside to enjoy its splendor which was showering light above the old dairy barn to the West. After a while he turned to head back to the house and in the Northern sky the largest comet that he had ever seen went flashing across the horizon. It was such a feeling of blissfulness to witness this moment, almost like time had ceased to exist. On November 7th, the alignment was causing an eclipse of the moon, an evening that was spent at Jim and Mary Jo's along with other family members, watching this moment unfold.

One-week later Fran and Traveler's twenty-six-year marriage and life together came to an end. Although peaceful and somber in nature the reality only set in a couple of weeks later. Traveler shared the news with Rory when he returned home from working in Ottawa and he said that just today he was sharing with his co-worker how rock solid his parents were as a couple and that they would be in it for the long haul. Rory said to his father, "This changes everything." Traveler knew what being an example meant, but life was bringing change, another fork in the road.

One evening shortly after they separated, he was sitting alone with their dogs at his feet looking around at the beauty of their home, the two-hundred-year-old pine floors, the three foot thick stone walls which had originally taken over five years to construct, and this modern kitchen seemingly etched from a magazine. This was the moment where the weight of Mother Earth came to rest on Traveler. His ego seemed to say "Traveler, look at all that you are leaving behind, the realization of a lifelong dream, your paradise to enjoy during those aging years and the place where your grandchildren will set their family roots." Oh yes, the feeling of whopped puppy stayed with him for the better part of an hour and then it was time to suck it up. Creator had never let him down, just needed to be open as to what was next for his journey.

Penny had passed away earlier that year after a short battle with cancer. Traveler's mother seemed to be able to manage a fair bit of pain without allowing it to affect her character. Penny had sensed the severity of her health problem in the Summer of 2002 but chose not to see a specialist, she preferred to hold off hearing this confirmation until later in the Fall. Traveler clearly remembers the moment she came into his office at the farm to give him a hug before leaving on vacation with Marlene and a friend.

The hug was different this time there was a sense of understanding and peacefulness in her touch, in her presence. It was like their souls shared the news. Traveler had prayed all of his life that his parents would have a long joyful stay here. He was hoping for a chance to grow up while they were still here to share their life experiences with him and his with them.

On the day of his mother's funeral as the family reached the Kinloch Road just passed his Parent's home; he took his foot of the gas pedal for a second or two wandering if anyone had stopped by to pick up Penny on the way through. Ah yes, she is no longer here. Although she would never give the family her real age throughout her life and took that truth with her at least in mind, she lived a wonderful 88 years. Her sister, Aunt Mary was well aware of her birth date but out of respect never shared the information. Father Calvin who Traveler's Parents loved and respected probably will have to bear a little karmic debt if Maggie has anything to say about it, as he divulged her true age at her farewell Mass. Many years have gone by since that day and there are times when Traveler would love to be able to sit at the kitchen table with her sharing a cup of tea and one of her homemade oatmeal-raisin cookies, over a heart-to-heart discussion on their lives. May she have realized her true Self before that last breath gave way to a continuing life eternal, ever dreaming, ever experiencing.

    By December first of that year and for the first time in his life, Traveler was moving into an apartment in the city to live alone, something he had never experienced. He viewed the move as the next level of non-attachment. Unknowingly it was the first step down a fork in the road where he would be travelling with less material things in his life. He furnished the two-bedroom apartment with his mother's bed and couch, a chair that he had used to meditate on at the farm and his computer complete with desk. It was an opportunity to continue his journey inward, Traveler knew deep down that this moment was a gift from Creator, a chance to move closer to Him. He continued to put life's learning into practice each moment of each day. He was trying to have absolute confidence in God while pondering on where life would lead him next. He felt, for the most part, peace and bliss in his life but there was still an underlying fear of shortage or lack of resources to survive. No matter how much income had come into his life in the past he was still dealing with shortage, never seemed to be enough. In reality, placing a clear vision in mind was easy, making a lavish image or dream big was the problem. Traveler did not have much interest in big boats, planes, a garage full of cars etc., the main reason for the vision was to create enough cash flow to be free, but the Universe does not flow with limitations. Traveler always felt that with enough cash-flow he would head for India or Thailand to search for a Spiritual teacher, but it was not to be.

    Fear in any form can only accumulate more fear and continually suck the life out of you. There are so many little negative or habitual patterns that have to be removed before encountering one's purpose here. It would take quite a few more years before Traveler had a handle on fear and lack of money. He would have to face his greatest fear of being without money.

He was never quite sure whether the adjustment to apartment living was more difficult for him or for Johnnie, his Basenji who made the move with him. Johnnie had never been without a fireplace since landing in Canada and he adorned fire, laying with his nose almost touching the flame. There was no doubt that his fur was close to igniting sometimes during his fireside naps. It was good to have Johnnie around as he was always so happy to see Traveler return to the apartment. He seemed to adapt to their city life and enjoyed daily runs of freedom down by the canal, close to the St. Lawrence River. Traveler used to hide in the tall grass when Johnnie strayed off too far, which was every time, and scare him when he would run back looking for Traveler. Ah… the little things in life, that bring joy to the heart.

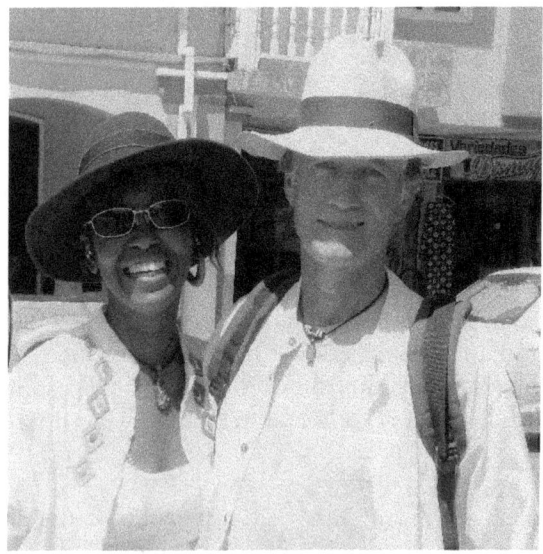

FINAL YEARS IN CANADA

Traveler received an email from Helga who lived in Toronto. She is another Lady whom he respected for her tenacity in life as she had become a successful Commercial Real Estate Agent while raising her daughter as a single Mother. Helga suggested that he meet her friend Gaby as she felt that they would have some common business interests and perhaps could work together for their mutual benefit. The timing was good as most other income streams for Traveler had come to a trickle. He contacted Gaby by email and within a couple of weeks they met in Toronto. Their discussions were on many things including a small Health Spa property in Costa Rica and other investment opportunities, but they soon discovered each other's passion for their spiritual journey.

They began to work together but there was always time spent sharing life's experiences and how they related to spirit. Traveler had heard of one particular Guru living in India back in 1999 during an event in Mexico, but never gave the name much attention. Gaby as it turned out, had been to India nine times to experience this Guru Sai Baba firsthand and had spent much time at his Ashram in Puttaparthi. Gaby would volunteer in whatever way she could. She had a deep love for Sai, something that Traveler did not totally understand at the time. It was the beginning of a relationship between Sai and Traveler, even though he never met him personally. Sai began to appear in Traveler's dreams which were normally lucid, quite real, and full of emotion. This contact in dreams spanned over four years and it was a little hard to perceive how this soul had a level of consciousness high enough to bring these dreams into play. It was about this time that Traveler began to learn more about the Hindu religion as well as Buddhism and this experience brought about a fairly big shift on his perception of many things in life, quite profound and beautiful.

Sai had said that all religions are a path leading back to God, one only needs to recognize the truth of his existence and stay on that path until he has reached a realization of Self. Sometimes words are spoken in a way to reach a person's level of understanding or consciousness so that they can take the best possible meaning or perception of this dialogue.

Religion(s) are founded on truth, whether it is a personal experience by the author, or an account of experiences written by a third party or witness. Where humanity normally takes a fork in their spiritual road is believing that their way is the best way or the only truth and stay on that road regardless of how it may have an effect on another person's truth. Later on, in this man's journey, the truth would begin to surface but not just yet, more to discover. At this point in his life his ego was getting ready to make a switch over to a spiritual person as the investment world was getting ready to deal the final blows. He did not really know that he had an ego and for sure did not realize that it was almost running his life…

There was one vision, memory, or connection to another time space that Traveler experienced in meditation during his stay in Toronto. He was in quiet time early in the morning when his consciousness went to an open field overlooking a small airport. It was the first time that Traveler felt his consciousness and senses together outside of this realm. He could feel the breeze as the tall grass was blowing in the wind, an older twin prop plane dated back to the late fifties, was landing on the nearby runway. Traveler was a short distance from a mountain Lion, perhaps 5 or 6 feet away. Traveler could see every aspect of this wild cat, shiny coat, his ears, and eyes and wondered if the animal could sense Traveler's presence. It was a profound experience, seem to overload his body's senses for the better part of the day. He had a breakfast meeting with Gaby that day and she understood the feeling as she had similar experiences during her life.

Their business ventures during that first year started out well and it looked very promising that cash-flow would be good. Traveler did a lot of driving during this time and enjoyed being on the road alone with just his thoughts, each phone call seem to be bringing more business and more gratitude for his life. Most of what was happening in these passing months were more of an illusion or the beginning of a bad dream, but he was unaware of this.

Before long promises from financial institutions were being delayed and eventually, they defaulted completely which would eventually lead to a point where investors were holding another piece of worthless paper for the fire. With each passing day it became more difficult to decipher the reality from the illusion. Each decision came with one more disappointment not only for Gaby and Traveler but for others who had hoped to capitalize on their participation. Each day brought with it a further need to search within for some sense of truth. Gaby and Traveler became leaning posts for each other as events unfolded and any hope of understanding the situation became almost impossible. It was not long into this saga that the real or hidden lives of some people involved came to light or perhaps darkness is a better description. There were at least four or five investors that had or previously had dealings with the suit and tie mafia, you would never know it by looking at them, only regular folk. They began to use threats up to a point of wanting to take the lives of the principal agent/person that had been successful in this particular business for over ten years. All of this was beginning to drive home the fact that there was little that was real in the investment world. Traveler had a hard time to understand the depth of attachment to money that many had, it could move them to a point of rage and a position that they would get their capital back at all costs. It was a wake-up call for Traveler, few people are who they appear to be, depending on the mask they are sporting for you. Who are we? There's a plan in place, one just needs to hold fast on the journey home until you take the time and effort to connect with your true Self.

It was during this tumultuous period of life that Traveler had made a move to the historic city of Brockville along the St. Lawrence. It was really like a break-out from living close to home all his life, it only took 48 years, no hurry. It was before he knew that the wheels were getting ready to fall off his business ventures. This charming city with a population of approximately fifty-five thousand is situated at the entrance of the Thousand Islands. It was founded by some of the wealthiest settlers to Canada and most of the castles and glorious stone homes remain today carrying their history forward.

Traveler was fortunate enough to find an apartment close to the river and the many beautiful walkways that this paradise has to offer. His apartment was part of a building that was originally owned by a local Judge. This home was built in a Victorian style which the new owners, David & Joan maintained in their theme while converting it into five apartments. The property also included a two-story living space called the Coach house along with beautiful gardens for all residents to enjoy. Johnnie immediately approved of the move to their fully furnished home which included a beautiful view of the river along with the site of many freighters and pleasure boats that travelled the waterway.

Traveler soon became acquainted with his neighbors and enjoyed the odd summer afternoon over an ale with Betty, Hurdie and Dianna along with Harry and Lynn. Traveler enjoyed this area immensely and it was far enough away from his home that he could begin to detach from a lifetime of memories. Charlotte and her boyfriend Josh came for a visit that Summer after a couple of months of tree planting in Northern Ontario. Rory would make the trip up to spend an evening with Traveler on one of the many boat cruises with Captain Andy. Traveler truly felt at home in this little gem of a city.

September brought a new resident to the building, would she fit in with the social group which now included Jim and Brenda from across the street. Within the first day or so it was clear that B was more than happy to share time with this group of friends, and it quickly became inevitable that she would be the social director. Wonderful… another being to share these precious times with.

Traveler was used to frequenting the local restaurants and dining alone but soon B was accompanying him and enhancing the experience. B's sparkling blue eyes emitted excitement, like a young soul looking to experience life's adventures with a deep passion. She has a natural enthusiasm in all that she does, something that Traveler often wanted more of in his life. Although he had enthusiasm and bliss flowing through his veins, his very essence, it didn't always show through in his quiet manner. Perhaps there was still some unknown weight on his heart that needed to be lifted.

They soon began to share their lives and almost all of their leisure time together. Jim and Brenda became close friends, and many evenings were spent around the dining room table sharing the week's events or just humorous stories and laughter.

Jim always had an endless resource of life's experiences to share, he was in the top ten standings for motorcycle drivers on the North American Racing circuit, so that covered a few years. One fine sunny morning Jim's mother was riding on the back of his motorcycle heading to their work. As usual Jim was clipping along at a fair pace when he suddenly ducked down to miss an oncoming bird. It was not long after and his mother was hitting him on his back with both hands. Jim couldn't figure out what was wrong, so he quickly pulled over to the side of the road. When he turned around to see if his mother was alright, he saw that she had the little bird stuck in her mouth, what a site.

Brenda has since left her mortal body after a short battle with cancer. Brenda was one of those incredibly special beings that had an inherent knowing of what was right and quietly worked her magic in caring for her community and those in need. Her presence in that city will long be remembered as will her efforts for the betterment of those who knew her.

Traveler's Father slipped away early December in 2004 while living in the retirement Manor, a place that became his home for the last few years of his life. As an observer it may have appeared to be an unfitting end for a man who was so vibrant during his active years and passionate about life, especially the education of youth in the area surrounding his birthplace and home. There is no easy way of knowing his relationship with his Creator while his body was under the grip of Parkinson's disease. The last time that Traveler spent visiting with his father, he was unable to speak, and his body had become very rigid, but there was still a deep expression of life coming from his clear blue eyes. Traveler wondered at that moment if perhaps his father was having some of his best communion with his Source.

When father Sam (seems like the name was fitting) was a high school student Sister Superior had asked him to become a priest, something Traveler's father had taken into consideration but did not accept. His father's journey was filled with many accomplishments, and anything written in these pages would pale in the reality of his story. His disease which robbed him of his physical strength and mobility quite possibly was induced by an incorrect diagnosis of prostate cancer by a well-meaning Doctor. Although Traveler's father was very much into Natural remedies he had grown up through an era where Doctors were looked upon as knowing all when it came to health issues. His father had followed the Doctor's advice and for 6 months he was committed to a medication that he could have lived without, his body weight dropped probably by almost 20 pounds or more. Most days when Traveler stopped over for a visit his father would be laying on the floor trying to gather strength but by the time he decided to discontinue the medication, the damage was done. He was given almost six months of renewed hope when a specialist started treating the disease that had now arisen as a result of the first drug doping treatment. Parkinson had brought the tremors and lack of mobility, the drugs to control this was the so-called renewed hope. Unfortunately, this Doctor/Specialist tried a mix of drugs to fine tune Sam's experience and he almost died from the lethal mix. Sam did make a partial recovery, but it became evident that he would not be able to return home and life as he had known it would never be quite the same. Sam and Penny's sixty years of life together was nearing an end, another fork in the road.

There is a story about Ramana Maharishi who as a boy of twelve or thirteen at the time and while in his bedroom one day, felt that he was going to physically die. He accepted the oncoming death and lay down on the bed to be a witness to his body slowly stop functioning almost in a mummified state until only his consciousness remained, and at that point realized his true eternal nature. Ramana's body regained its life, but he knew that it would be impossible to share this reality with his family, so he left his home and soon became one of the most recognized Sages in India. Perhaps father Sam experienced that state of consciousness during his final days in the retirement home.

On the day of his Father's funeral, arrangements had been made to have the precession drive by the Public School which had been named after him, in honor of his dedication to education during forty-seven years of his life. All of the young students stood lined up in front of the school to say their last goodbye to a man they had come to love and respect. Sam's farewell Mass was given at his home Parish of Glenevis during a cold blistery day in December. Art who was Sam's closest ally on the School Board and over the years had become his best friend was asked to give the eulogy. For sure Art had shed a few tears prior to this day as he prepared to share a few highlights of his friend's life with those in attendance. In perfection Art recapped Sam's life and bid him farewell. May the pipes play on in memory of that day as Sam was laid to rest beside Penny, may their beautiful souls play on in another space and time...

As the months progressed, B and Traveler enjoyed many wonderful times together and became supportive of each other's lives. He continued his focus on Self-discovery and B showed a genuine interest in her search for the truth, each one experiencing their own truth in their own way... Although many of his life's experiences may have seemed unreal to B, she never doubted the validity of them and was always open to hearing more. Deep inside Traveler knew that at some point again in his life he would have to journey alone, becoming more separated from the world at least for a while.

It was during this time that Traveler signed up for a course in Ottawa to learn more about the Merkaba field and the meditation practice to initiate the Merkaba and maintain its rotation. There was one exercise that the Instructor had the small class try before getting into the mechanics of the Merkaba. Each person had a partner and sat knee to knee in front of each other, the closer the better and stared into each other's eyes for at least ten minutes. This is definitely uncomfortable for most people including Traveler as they all feel that they have something to hide. In reality there is nothing about life that a person needs to feel shame or guilt about. As Traveler focused on the other person's eyes, they eventually changed color and were the eyes of a wild animal, similar to a Lion. Each one in the class had a unique experience as they shared what they saw, some had a complete face change. It is a good exercise for couples to look into the beyond…

Their lives were changing, and this mutual support became all important, perhaps part of the plan. With each passing month, life's tests were taking their toll on Traveler. He had come to enjoy life by the river immensely and if times were different, he would definitely consider making this area his permanent home. The reality of a year of effort being completed with little income was trying and it eventually became inevitable that any promised payment would not be forthcoming. Traveler had leaned on his family all too much during that time and once again Mother Earth was hovering outside the window waiting for a decision.

Traveler had often talked to Rod about living in Ecuador and he would jokingly send an email or call once in a while asking when he would be coming down to enjoy the never-ending Spring weather. Traveler had visited Rod and his wife in the beginning of 2004 and saw the natural beauty of this small country. Traveler was swaying towards a move but not enough yet to detach him from life in the Thousand Islands.

One can enjoy all things that this world has to offer and allow the senses to experience life to the fullest but on this so-called spiritual journey of life, it appears necessary to remove any attachment to it, just enjoy it as it presents itself. Traveler knew the feeling all too well that was beginning to swell up inside of him, like a river rising from the Spring rain. Change was coming and he knew that a decision would have to be made shortly. It was a major fork in the road, but this time he could see it in the distance and prepare a bit for the turn.

THE CALL TO ECUADOR

Traveler made the call to Rod on a Monday morning after a restless night of sleep or lack of it. Rod was on his way to work so they had time to chat. He had been living in Ecuador for close to two and a half years and with his experience it would allow for an easier transition for Traveler to start a new life experience. Traveler had experienced a few countries in Central America and always felt that he would like to live in Latin America at some point, perhaps renovating old homes or building new ones but Creator had a different plan… This day was one of the longest of his life as he prepared to tell B of his decision.

Johnnie had sensed a change and was sticking to Traveler like glue that day, always there for morale support. Although Traveler was always emotionally soft on the inside it rarely came to the surface but as he shared that moment with B his heart became heavy, and his emotions could not be held back. It would be wonderful to journey through life without hurting another human being but perhaps impossible.

There were many things affecting his day, the thought of leaving Canada, the comfort and enjoyment of living by the river and his life experience with B and their friends. The other small detail was what kind of work would Traveler be doing. He is grateful to B for putting any sense of selfishness aside and decide to simply enjoy the time they had together. Being angry at another person for seemingly taking something away from their life is a common reaction but allowing freedom to another soul is an uncommon character strength.

As the reality set in, it was time to make plans and share his decision with Rory and Charlotte along with friends and family. Rory's make up perhaps was similar to Traveler when he was Rory's age, and there was no doubt that he would have preferred to have him within driving distance. It was always nice to be able to have an around the kitchen table chat every once in a while, a time of sharing that Traveler had always had with his parents. Charlotte had lived away from their home for almost five years and saw the adventure of this move. They all agreed that they were only a flight away from each other, but little did they know that it would be a couple of years before they'd see each other.

How to prepare for a move to another country with no resources in hand, yes it certainly presents a challenge. Once again with the help of family and friends, Traveler had enough money to plan for his move South. He was originally going to leave from home and head directly to Ecuador, but Rory and Charlotte were kind enough to pay for his flight to Vancouver so that they could share some time together before he headed out. Trying to make decisions in life with no money was something that Traveler was not accustomed to. There is a difference between having a little and having none. What did life have in store for Traveler? It was exciting and frightening all in one energy and it seemed like he was being pushed into the fork in the road rather than making a decision.

There were not many things in his possession at that time, but it was surprising how much Traveler had to get rid of in order to pack the remainder of his life's belongings into 3 bags. The exercise did not allow for much attachment to anything material, just a few memories. There were boxes of books that went to the Used Book Store in Town and a few other family treasures that were left behind with his sister and brother Jim.

He had read many stories on people giving up their wealth to devote their life to God in hope of realizing the truth of their existence. Traveler understood the concept, but he could honestly say that he was apprehensive about truly living it. He still had that little fear of shortage, and you may wonder how that could be possible.

Fear does not go away on its own, firstly one needs to find out where this energy is arising from. That perhaps is the first step and then it is a matter of clearing or releasing these memories. Somewhere along this road you will discover that the propaganda initiated by our governments, is being sent out every second of the day through media and much of this subliminal programming is designed to keep the human race in fear.

What are we afraid of? Many are feeling some kind of shame or guilt of something that happened in their past, others have a feeling of never being good enough and are concerned about losing their job or their relationships. Bringing the past up every day in our conversations and thoughts only keeps us trapped in the past, never allowing ourselves to start out fresh today, creating this new and wonderful you. At some point, if you continue on this wisdom path to the truth, you will let go of the past and put all of your trust in your Source. How could it be any other way than allowing That which created you, to provide for you. Your right, it is not that easy but at some point, you will be required to at least, begin to let go.

Traveler was so grateful for the opportunity to spend time with Rory and Charlotte before the move to Ecuador. He felt more like the child leaving the nest and they were there for morale support. Their maturity and love shone through and gave him strength to journey on. He had been blessed with much travel in his life but stepping away from his homeland long-term was a new experience.

Charlotte dropped him off in Squamish to take the bus back into Vancouver and other than riding in a bus for sports events or social activities, Traveler had never really taken a bus to go from point A to point B. It would be the first of many bus rides that he was about to experience in Ecuador. It was back to Ontario to spend an evening with Marlene before she dropped him off at the Airport the following day. Once again, the feeling was that of a young boy leaving home. It's funny how after a few thousand lifetimes and almost fifty years into this one, he could still feel like a child.

Rod was kind enough to have the VIP service waiting for Traveler at the Airport in Quito and avoid the long line-ups through the immigration process. It was perhaps one more opportunity for the little ego to breathe life, but it would be short lived.

Rod and his wife are always gracious hosts, and they had their guest Cabaña ready for his stay. Traveler's first couple of weeks were spent as a tourist, enjoying all the beauty that Ecuador has to offer. It was also a time to enjoy Rod and Pierrette's company along with that of their son Allan and his family who had been living in Ecuador during the past six months.

Allan was teaching English in Quito at the time and was preparing to leave that job to work alongside Rod at a new construction project. Within a couple of weeks Traveler replaced Allan at the Institute and began teaching English. Yes, your memory is correct, he did not have any teaching experience but teachers with a native tongue being English were in demand, especially in the larger cities of Ecuador. He still had not quite conquered being comfortable walking back from communion, but it was time for a little stretch of self-confidence with a classroom full of students.

Over the next week or so Allan showed him the ropes on riding the bus from Cumbaya to Quito and arrive at the school within an hour. He spent about three days sitting in on a few classes and by the end of the week, he was a teacher or at least he had the teaching manuals, a dictionary, and a key to his locker. Allan was kind enough to lend Traveler his translator which was a God sent, especially for those students who were in the beginning levels of learning English.

Soon he was into the routine of riding the bus back and forth into the city. Every day was a new experience one that Traveler enjoyed immensely. Most days the buses were packed with commuters which ranged from businesspeople to local Indigenous (Quechua) who were heading into Quito to sell their products. It is a different experience to be part of the culture rather than seeing it as a tourist. Each day the bus transported products ranging from prize roosters to pails brimming with strawberries. Traveler kept wondering how he could experience all of this for twenty-five cents. On a normal day, the bus ride into Quito is almost thirty minutes long and only cost a quarter. There are spectacular views as you journey out of the valley in Cumbaya and chug along up the highway. From the base of the valley to the mountain ridge where Quito begins is a climb of about five hundred meters, with the magical view changing around every curve.

On a clear day Cotopaxi stands alone with its snowcapped peak and usually a glimpse of Cayambe and Antisana the other two volcanoes that expose their beauty around the city of Quito. He enjoyed, in perhaps a small way, being part of this

Ecuadorian culture and seeing how they approach each day, many with laughter and optimism of a better day tomorrow. Traveler still had a good amount of optimism and confidence in his being, from days gone by and somehow felt a sense of what their journey entailed.

Although the rate of four dollars an hour seems like quite a cut in pay for teaching, it probably was considered a middle-class salary for Ecuador at that time. It is relevant to the cost of living there which is unbelievably low in comparison to Canada or the United States. After Traveler got over the fear of standing up in front of a few students in class, he began to enjoy them. It was a wonderful opportunity to meet people who were working with the United Nations or Diplomats from Embassies in Quito as well as Military personal and High School students. It was a pleasure to be able to share their life stories and their vision of the future and of course answer all their questions about Canada. All of the teachers were great to work with and were always helpful when Traveler had any questions on the course material. These teachers were from many different countries including the United States, Venezuela, Romania, Canada, England, and Ecuador.

As it appeared that he would be able to teach for a while, he found an apartment close to the school and about a ten-minute bus ride away from the office where Rod was working. Traveler's apartment had a rooftop deck with a beautiful view of the city and the surrounding Volcanoes. Rod and Pierrette were kind enough to lend a dresser and night tables along with a few other necessities so that Traveler could be on his own again, almost independent. He was now able to return to a disciplined routine of meditation and focus on the narrow path searching for his truth.

Traveler had made a promise to Creator, over the past couple of years, that when he moved to South or Central America, he would begin to volunteer or be of service somehow.

When a promise is made, especially to your Creator, it is important to be loyal to your Self and follow through with your commitment.

Not long after his move to Quito the thought came to look for an Orphanage and so the search began. You would think that it would be an easy task, but it took a little effort. He began to ask his students and finally one of them who was a Nurse, knew of an Orphanage in the old historic city of Quito in an area called Recoleta. On a Saturday morning Traveler hopped on the trolley bus and headed South and during the trip a woman sitting next to him confirmed that he was on the right bus and indicated which (Parada) Stop to get off. He arrived in Recoleta after about a forty-minute ride, seemed simple enough. Traveler began walking up and down the streets asking locals, in his limited Spanish where the Orphanage was located, nobody had heard of any, but eventually a Policeman directed him back down the street to a Church. Traveler rapped on the large wooden doors until one of the resident Sisters finally appeared, but she just shook her head, probably out of misunderstanding. She said that he should come back tomorrow and speak with el Padre. He stepped back into the street and said to Creator "You will have to make it a little easier than this if we are going to find the location, perhaps a sign of some kind."

Recoleta is one of the poorer neighborhoods in the city, so he was not all that anxious to wonder up and down every street. Traveler walked up to the end of one street and turned right, within thirty seconds he began to see signs with Niños (children) on them and sensed that he was heading in the right direction. Down the street on a large stone archway there was a sign that read St. Vincent de Paul and soon he was standing at the gate calling out "Bueños dìas." It was not long before Traveler was speaking with Sister Emma, who was the Mother Superior for the Orphanage, fortunately she could understand a bit of English. She soon had Lindsey an American student who was the head of volunteers, translating for them. After that conversation between Sister Emma and Lindsey, it was agreed that he would return in July and begin his formal training in order to help out in some way.

Traveler's first thoughts about volunteering were the possibility of teaching English to the classes that were held at the Orphanage, but the classes were out for summer break. Sister Emma was concerned about his lack of Spanish speaking skills, rightly so. He said that he could help out in the kitchen if necessary, but Sister Solara was very protective of her kitchen, so he began his Sunday mornings working with about fifteen children between the ages of one and a half to two years old. Almost always American students would get them bathed and dressed for the day and bring them into the playroom one by one.

Traveler was there to keep them entertained and share his love or more accurately experience theirs. These little treasures could rip a hole in your heart rather quickly as he began to see their personalities shine through. As in any group setting there is usually a pecking order, and it was interesting to see how each child dealt with the daily rigors of life. Juan liked to work in silence to keep up his image as the tough guy. He never had a mean look about him but would just calmly walk over to one of the children and take their toy or just a little shove to knock them of balance. Maria was a solid little girl with hair that sprang out in every direction, and she always smiled through every aspect of her face. Maria was probably the real leader in the group as Juan rarely went near her unless it was in the nature of sharing. Sebastian was a firecracker usually running on his toes at top speed until somebody tripped him or the wall jumped out to slow him down. In the first couple of months, he cried quite often and demanded a lot of attention, but he gradually changed into a quiet young lad, hmm not sure how that happened.

It was normally the same routine on Sunday where all the children were taken outside, to spring them loose in the back lawn to burn off some energy. The first Sunday was a beautiful warm day so Sister Solara decided it would be a good day to erect the swimming pool. Out of the diapers and into their swimming trunks, there was so much excitement as they all piled into the water. It was amazing to watch because they all played and splashed each other without a tear.

It was time to drain the pool and put it away for another day. As the children ran around in total freedom, they were slowly rounded up to get dressed and inside for their lunch. It was the same lunch every day, a very thick soup and one by one they were fed. This day was a challenge as the fresh air and water play had worn them out. From the table to the crib for a nap and by that time Traveler was ready for a nap himself. Maybe it was a combination of adjusting to the altitude of Quito at twenty-seven hundred and fifty meters and of course the time spent running after the children.

He looked forward to each coming Sunday as he had grown fond of them. Each day at the Orphanage brought many wonderful memories. Soul seemed to be drawn to Traveler and most days would fall asleep in his lap. His twin sister Carlita was a beautiful girl who always seemed to be self-amused never bothering anyone and never being bothered. These siblings along with three or four other children eventually moved into La Casa in another part of the Orphanage, where they could become part of a family setting, it was wonderful to see the transition as their characters changed a bit. In the family setting they seemed to be able to drop any protective barrier that they might have carried. Things can be a little rough in the Orphanage as patience runs thin.

Jose was about as big as a minute and loved having Traveler swing him in the air to kick a ball with his feet. He only had one speed which was wide open and was so full of life and energy. Traveler nick named him butterfly boy as he was infatuated with them. The butterflies felt the attraction and as soon as he would see one his eyes would light up and soon, they would be on his hand or floating around him, it was magic to watch. On the other hand, there was Sebastian who was terrified of them and would shake as he ran for safety. Jose fell asleep on Traveler's lap or near him every Sunday before lunch. They all seem to look for a place to rest but Jose usually dropped like a stone after play time.

Ana was another child whose presence was evident as she was quite petite in stature, but she was another one that was rarely bothered by any of the other children. Her smile was infectious as it never waned. She soon became a regular along with a few others to curl up in Traveler's arms for a little break before lunch. Some days he wandered if being there was really making a difference or whether he was only there trying to perform penance of some sort. He tried to put it into a larger perspective comparing it to his own life. Could it be for that brief moment Ana somehow felt absolute peace in her heart, with no fear or no need to protect herself from the other children. Perhaps she could for a moment feel love and radiate that peaceful love that was flowing in her heart. Traveler soon realized that these days of sharing their lives was as much for him as it was for Ana and the other precious souls, life rolling along in chaotic perfection.

Over the next few months these Sunday trips to Recoleta continued and one day once again Traveler was questioning the purpose of him being there, ah yes… a little down day. It was lunch time and after feeding a couple of children one of them was giving him some grief by not wanting to eat, so one of the volunteers knew the routine and asked to switch places with her.

Traveler hadn't seen this young boy before, but he suspected that the little lad was just being introduced to the group. As he looked at his smiling face surrounded by this afro style abundance of hair, he couldn't help but smile. He continued to feed him and with each bite he would slowly slide

Journey Home

into his chair almost falling asleep but never losing his smile. By this time, he was attracting the attention of the other volunteers along with Sister Solara and they began to laugh. Sister smiled and gave Traveler the signal that it was time to take him to his crib. Each child has their name above the crib, but Traveler could not understand the name she was calling him so one of the workers came along to point out the right crib. Isaid is his name and his smile helped to take Traveler out of his moment of despair or maybe more correctly bring him back to the moment…

There is no doubt that it can be difficult for the human mind to grasp the immensity and beauty of Creation, not to be discouraged, our mind is not capable of perceiving It, but we can become more aware of Its presence. If we were constantly being aware of the presence of spirit in our life, that would be a refreshing start, but our ego/mind becomes so programmed during our lifetime that it is almost totally caught up somewhere else, planning for the future. Waking up and at least becoming interested in the journey home is a great start to coming into alignment with this wisdom path that will open up your truth. Breath is always one sure way to become aware, Drunvalo calls this action "conscious breathing". While you breathe just pause the breath as you inhale or exhale and immediately you are in the present, connected to Source. If you can practice this breathing from time to time the blissful moments will eventually turn into blissful days. While living in gratitude you can begin to experience the loving presence of Spirit each day and truly witness miracle after miracle unfolding in your life.

One beautiful sunny Sunday, Traveler got off the trolley bus and while walking back to his apartment, questions began to arise. He was living on the equator far away from Canada his home for almost fifty years, but he was experiencing no difference here as he looked around and felt very much at home in Quito. He began to ask questions about being there, teaching, volunteering, and living on his own, seemed to be insignificant whether he was living on Mother Earth or not. Traveler believes that as one becomes more aware or conscious, they begin to question many things about the world that they are experiencing each day. If the search is for Truth, then ultimately one will have to look inward, where the mystery will be revealed.

Traveler was nearing his apartment and as was quite common to see at many intersections in the city, a young boy was pushing his father in a wheelchair. They made their trek up and down the hill between the cars looking for a little kindness to help them through another day. The man in the wheelchair was without arms and legs but even with this disability he continually smiled at each and every person that caught his gaze whether they reached out to help or not. Traveler thought to himself; what is the real purpose of this daily routine, other than the obvious need to survive… He continued to look out from his apartment window as the father and his son continued up the hill only to roll back down and start over with the next group of cars. This man's smile never deviated and always a nod of the head in gratitude to those that shared.

Maybe the man in the wheelchair was a gift to his son so he could experience at a young age the true sense of giving of himself, perhaps it was not only about the father's disability. Another perspective was that his son was not only building his physical body with the constant effort of pushing his father up the hill, but he was also developing his character strength inside as he witnessed the emotion of each passing person. How would his experience have a ripple effect as the boy's presence influenced others, those other individuals that cried about their difficulties in life. Traveler had his answers for today, it was time to relax and enjoy the rest of the day.

Since arriving in Ecuador and before that time, Traveler had thought about exporting products back into Canada. It seemed like a good opportunity to benefit not only themselves but the manufacturers or Artists of these products. Allan had similar thoughts and soon Saturday afternoons at Rod and Pierrette's became the place for master minding and creating the vision of the potential for this venture. Traveler's mind was still working with the power of thought although it may not have been fully functional after the events that had passed in Canada, nevertheless he stayed focused on creating once again with the elixir of faith and living in gratitude.

In the beginning, everywhere they looked seem to offer the opportunity to export for profit as different products presented themselves. Rod being the more conservative one tried to keep things in perspective, but they all enjoyed talking about the possibilities. They began to focus on construction material as it was an area that they had a little expertise in and during that time the Canadian economy was strong with a continuing building boom. After much discussion, they narrowed the search down and focused on finding quality ceramic tile and hardwood flooring. Within a few months of searching, travelling and meetings they finally had a product that would appeal to the Canadian market coupled with a price competitive with products coming out of China at that time.

By November, after many barbecues at Rod's they had their first order for product. This company that had fit all criteria was located in Cuenca so Allan and Traveler decided that it would be best if he moved to Cuenca to monitor shipments and help with logistics from manufacturer to destination port. On Christmas Eve Allan and his family, along with Traveler's worldly possessions loaded in the back of the Jimmy, were heading to Cuenca. This city built high in the Andes has a history dating back almost five hundred years. There are three rivers that flow through the city giving it an undeniable special energy that you can feel upon your arrival. It is the gem of Ecuador and has become a popular destination for expats.

Traveler had another teaching job in place and had found a family to live with who were located in the historic center of

Cuenca. He wanted to live with a local family while taking Spanish lessons to try and master the language or at least be able to communicate in it. Cuenca is located in the mountains at an altitude of 2,500 meters and of all the places that he had seen in Ecuador to date it was one of the most beautiful places to live. Cuencanos are proud of their heritage that has been influenced by the Spaniards and Indigenous people. It is known as the cultural center of Ecuador as many of the Country's Poets, Writers and Artists are from there and it continues that prestigious title today. His host family's Father was a well-known Doctor in the city as well as a Philosopher and Author. This move to Cuenca was an easy transition and Traveler enjoyed all that it had to offer.

Allan and he spent a few hours at the manufacturing plant on the twenty-seventh to witness their first two containers being loaded and sealed for their destination to Vancouver. It was a great feeling after almost eight months of effort. Allan and his family headed back to Cumbaya the next morning and Traveler began to settle into his new surroundings. In Cuenca there seem to be a parade or festival most weekends and over the Christmas celebration there was one almost every day right through the month of January. Since the English Institute was closed for the holidays, Traveler had time to check out the sites, meet the locals and of course find a few restaurants.

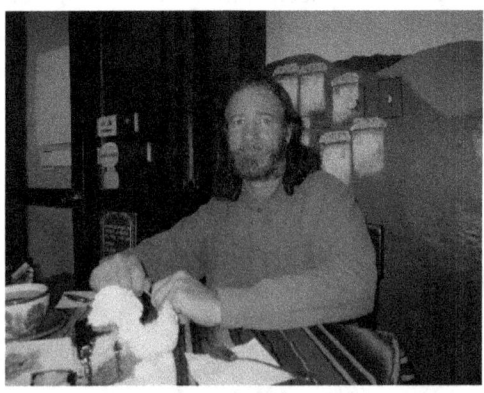

MAHABHARATA

Over the past year Traveler had been aware of and studied a bit of the teachings of the Gita. The teachings of the Bhagavad Gita are widely accepted, especially in the Hindu spiritual community, as a guide to righteous living and conduct in order to attain freedom and return to the Truth of existence. Gita is small part of a grand story called Mahabharata. Part of this wisdom within these teachings were taught to Arjuna over 5000 years ago by Krishna who was an Avatar on Earth. It is said that Krishna's mission was to re-establish dharma or righteousness within humanity once again. These teachings were hidden or lost from mankind over different periods of our time on Earth but are here in this Age to help one to remember our potential or awaken to It.

Traveler was now studying these teachings for at least one or two hours each day and trying to implement them into his daily activities. He was now becoming aware of another level of surrender far beyond his previous comprehension of its meaning; while lying on the hood of the car in Kentucky. This mind which had been his tool in creating, through holding a thought or vision was no longer to be used in that capacity, at least not until Traveler had a complete understanding of its connection to Source. There was confusion as he wondered about letting go of this learned science and the seeming abundance that it brought into his life. He had heard of times called the dark period of the soul and wondered if this was such a time. Oh... not yet, not even close. He felt blessed every day just to be aware of these teachings and to have the time in his life to study and be alone. As each day went on, he realized the power of the mind or more correctly the power that he had handed over to it, unconsciously. Our soul takes on the experience of the human body in its natural state of peace, purity, and innocence as all of this is its true nature. Mahabharata speaks of karmic debt that is within the DNA of the chosen body which can become a point of ignorance or darkness (dense energy) as the soul slowly forgets its eternal connection with Source. Our body (normally chosen in the same lineage as a previous lifetime) and mind continue to receive programming from an outside source (parents, schools, government, media etc.) turning the mind's focus on the outside world. Hence the necessity to wake up... It takes effort to break old habits and heal old memories but that is our responsibility during each lifetime that we experience here. It is a time at present where many truths are coming into the light or into plain site for each one of us, to assist us in living free in knowing.

By the middle of January Traveler was well settled into his routine of teaching and also learning Spanish each day Monday through Friday. He continued to study the information contained in the Gita and tried to implement these teachings into his daily life. It was now time for the next level of commitment on his journey. He decided that the next morning in meditation he would once again surrender this human experience to his Creator, but certainly with a different understanding of what this meant. As more knowingness and understanding comes into your life experience so does a shift in consciousness.

How does one surrender their life to God? That is a really good question and Traveler thought that he had the answer at this time. It seemed that the mind was the problem at least in its working capacity in Traveler's life at this juncture. The mind seldom stopped its never-ending flow of thoughts, always taking him away from the present moment. This was the mind that was creating visions to co-create here on Earth, that wasn't quite accurate, but Traveler would have to live with that perception for a while.

What Traveler really wanted to do was to surrender, he was relatively happy and content but still feeling a little heavy in the heart. He wanted to give this mind and all of its thoughts back to Source, let Him guide Traveler from here on in, take life as it came rather than all this planning and tension that too many thoughts can create. It takes a significant amount of trust to give it all over to Father/Mother, the ego does not give up its position easily, something that would take a few more years to understand. Hold Fast… It was definitely a walk in the dark, but Traveler was willing to experience whatever came his way and live it. From the doer to the observer, Traveler had read it a number of times but really… how does that work.

His life in Cuenca was enjoyable, no denying that, but there were many times that he was down to his last dollar or a less. He still had an attachment to eating and some days a banana and a 50-cent ice cream looked pretty shinny. The mind and ego continued to cause a bit of havoc and every once in a while, would try and take Traveler back to the so-called better days such as having a bed that he needed to get on his tip toes to get in to, now the floor was only 8 or 9 inches from his pillow. Many times, he would see a family enjoying the moment as they were driving down the street in their new car. Mind was quick to bring Traveler back to such moments in Canada, but just as quickly he would take himself back to the present and know that he was on the right track. Creator had never let him hit ground. Traveler didn't need to walk very far before coming upon other souls sleeping on a piece of cardboard huddled with their family on an abandoned veranda. It would make his almost empty apartment look pretty upscale in comparison.

Traveler was not looking for a quick fix, he wanted eternal happiness while living on Mother Earth, not a happiness that comes from the moment when you buy a new car or receive a good chunk of change to ease life's pain for a while. He was looking for something more permanent and was ready to put it all in, to experience it.

It's kind of like, don't try this at home folks, but not really. Each soul has his/her own journey ahead of them and it depends on the adventure that their higher Self is wanting to experience here. There is more but Traveler would come upon that later. The soul acts as the double for this higher Essence, which has many other experiences on other planes and then the unfoldment of this soul is within the body/mind/emotion here on this physical plane. The goal is for higher Self (Thought Adjuster) to integrate into this body and experience life through your awakening consciousness. The body/mind has to go through some major changes before that is possible.

Traveler needed to become mindless, well he had done that while drinking a bottle of Scotch a time or two, but this time required a more sustained effort. Quieting the mind might be a better description, pulling yourself back to the present until it begins to spend more time in spirit. Meditation each morning is like going to the pumps to fill up and prepare for the day ahead. There were not many down days where he wanted to through in the towel but there were moments where he wondered if he was on the right path or was he lost. Who are you going to call?

Traveler was never quite sure if it is all a bit of trial and error, but he suspected that God and Soul are playing the parts in perfection. Traveler was trying to give one meal a day to someone that he felt drawn to. He wasn't trying to play God just maybe make a difference in one person's life for a moment. He was trying to share while being neutral, but the bliss always flowed in when the expression of gratefulness beamed out from the less fortunate being. Giving seems to be more about receiving, can't stop it, call it love or Great Spirit, but it flows.

One Sunday as Traveler was heading into his most frequented restaurant for a meal that cost $1.10, he noticed an older gentleman standing on the street just off the curb, with a steel cane in hand. He was wearing a poncho and had a fairly nice sombrero (hat) on his head. Although his face was well tanned & weathered a bit, his stature was erect showing no real despair. Traveler wondered about offering him a meal but didn't want to offend him, so he greeted him and went inside to eat. While he was eating, he was still thinking about this gentleman and whether or not he was looking for something to eat. He finished up his lunch and walked back outside and this time Traveler noticed the man's small curled hand slightly out beyond the poncho signaling for help.

Traveler's Spanish speaking skills were no hell, but he managed to ask him if he would like a meal which he responded with a smile and a nod. He realized then how frail this man was as he helped him up onto the sidewalk and carried his plastic carrying case inside for him. Traveler arranged a meal for him and the waitresses inside were kind enough to set him up at a table.

As Traveler walked down the sidewalk, he gave gratitude for the moment and then as he was stepping onto the street there in front of him was a one dollar bill stuck up against the curb. It is a rare occasion to find money on the street in Ecuador and there might be a better chance of winning a lottery. Traveler accepted el dinero with gratitude and a feeling that at least for the moment he was perhaps on the right path. Traveler had many opportunities since that day to share a meal with Señor Lorenzo Manuel who shared many memories of better days gone by. Lorenzo had lost his three children and his wife a few years back and had to try and make it on his own with no pension to speak of, probably less than $100 a month or so that the government pension would provide him.

Where does one begin to live that love or permit that love which flows so naturally from Source? So close yet so far, what's holding it back? Traveler was in quiet time or meditation one morning when he had a profound experience, it appeared to be a laser beam of light coming from within, slowly burning off the layers of his body around his heart exposing its brilliance and then continuing in a circular fashion until the front of his body and head were gone. It was such a feeling of lightness without the weight of this inert matter pulling him down. The beam of light then went out into eternity, into the nothingness. Yes… the mind is a wonderful thing but eventually one begins to experience his own truth, who we really are, perception ever changing with each moment.

Now, who do you share your experiences with? Not everyone will believe you or even try to understand your enthusiasm, after all get serious, the real world is here on top of the pavement. There are very few within family or friends that will share a person's so called spiritual journey, most are interested in what is going on at work or what the weekend will bring and that is alright. In reality the experience here on Earth is yours and yours to unfold. Those who are on similar paths will pass through your life, some will stay for a while, and some will continue on their way. Truth will find Its way to you if you are looking, and at some point in your journey you will be required to speak Truth, if you agree to. It will flow out of you ready or not.

LIFE IN CUENCA

Traveler was continuing to experience the beauty of Ecuador and would make as many short trips as finances would permit. Jose was a young Lad who worked at the English School in Cuenca where Traveler was teaching. He invited Traveler to his family farm up in the mountains near Bucay, not only to meet his family but to help them with their idea to expand their little hog operation. He made the trip with Jose and his brother Giovani down into the coastal area and then back to the foothills heading towards Bucay.

Jose was thinking of returning to the farm to live and in order to realize that dream they needed to move forward with expansion, sounded familiar. They arrived at the base of the mountain where Jose's father was going to meet them with the horses, but they were a little early for the rendezvous, so they hopped in the back of a neighbor's pick-up truck and rode up the mountain for about fifteen minutes. Once the three of them had thanked the neighbor for the lift, they began to walk until they came to a point in the road that crossed a mountain path, Jose said that they would wait there for their ride.

There is beauty in almost every direction that you look in Ecuador and this mountain area was no different. Being in the coastal mountains feels like Summer in Canada, warm breeze, and blue skies. Within a few minutes Jose Sr. along with two saddled horses and a colt wandering behind, came out from a path through the trees. So, this was their mode of transportation on the next leg of their journey.

Jose and Traveler were the chosen ones and were fortunate enough to ride the horses up to the farm. As they climbed the mountain road each corner unfolded another scene of tranquility. There was a beautiful view of the valley unfolding below and off to the Southwest was a gateway between 2 mountains that led out to the thousands of hectares of lush farmland bountiful with bananas, rice and sugarcane extending all the way to the Pacific and the most populated city of Ecuador which is Guayaquil.

They passed through a little village called La Playa (The Beach) and Traveler thought that this was a strange name but later that day it became evident why it was called that. As the four travelers left the valley behind them, soon it was only the sound of streams flowing down the mountainside and melodies from songbirds courting them along. There were welcoming blue winged butterflies, big as a bird, appearing as their guides. Traveler asked Jose what the name of his horse was and after a bit of laughing his father confirmed that it had no name. That was the beginning of the song by America repeating in his mind for the next hour and a half. "A horse with no name." La la la la la la....

After a two hour ride, they arrived at the Hacienda not all that far from the peak of the mountain. They were greeted by Jose's mother Maria and his sister Adeli, as they toured the home Jose's family had built twenty-three years prior. There was a little stream flowing past the house that seemed to bring them to a timeless moment. Their kitchen was a small adobe shack standing alone on the hill behind the house. It had a grass (paja) roof which was covered with moss and white and purple wildflowers. Smoke was seeping out from the gable end assuring all that lunch was being prepared. As they ducked their heads down to step inside, it was like a step back in history. This dirt floor had been freshly swept, the only furniture was an old wooden table crowding the corner, where planks served as a seating area for those who were ready to eat or just share a story. Of course, the warmth that every country kitchen hold was enhanced with a wood burning fireplace where all family meals are prepared. A primitive fireplace yet served the purpose, even a flat rock jutting out from the foundation of the shack seemed perfect for the Tom Cat who was fast asleep on this perch, unaffected by the flames. Perhaps he was a distant relative of his African cousin, the Basenji race.

Shortly after their arrival fresh green Achira leaves filled the table as Adeli and her mother began to roll up the Quimbolita's for their treat later that afternoon. If there was a place on this Mother Earth where time had stopped it existed here on Jose's Hacienda. As in days gone by, most of the time spent for these women was in preparing meals.

That night they all slept in the small farmhouse, basically a few homemade wooden beds each complete with a thin mattress and a blanket or two. It was there that Traveler experienced darkness, couldn't see his hand, not even up close. He wasn't afraid of mice or rats when he was young, but somewhere along the way he developed a fear of these furry critters. Could have been the story about the rat that jumped at his grandfather's throat or the one where the little mouse ran up his Aunt Donelda's dress, somewhere along the way there was a shift. Traveler was fast asleep when he felt what he sensed was a little movement on the bed near his head. This is where the mind gets active rather quickly. The first re-action was to leap out of bed, but the darkness caused a moment of reflection, he had seen a kitten or two before going to bed, ah... yes that is the fur that he felt.

The next morning was a quick shave in front of the old car mirror hanging on the post holding up the porch. Before long breakfast was served and then out for a walk up the mountain. Traveler heard a little commotion amongst the chickens as they were leaving and suspected that one had been selected to join them for lunch. It was up the mountain where he witnessed the beauty below, the clouds had rolled in just below Las Playas and reached out to the sea giving it an appearance of a huge snow-white valley, spectacular. The boys made it back home in time for lunch, and as they stepped into the Kitchen, it was confirmed, the legs of the chicken were straight up interfering with the soup pot cover.

The following morning at four o'clock they were heading down the mountain road in a livestock truck carrying a few hogs, it was the only ride to the valley. On his trip back to Cuenca, Traveler was reflecting on these past few days. Where does he fit into this transformation on Mother Earth, on one side there was little change in the country life of Ecuador, on the other side there were the cities where Ecuadorian's were anxiously entering into middle class living. The banks where lending more money at this time, just like what had happened in Canada over 40 years before. Traveler had left Canada in part to get away from this fast pace of life and Ecuador seemed to offer this, but it was changing quickly. What was being grown organically here, which was an attraction for his style of living, was soon being sprayed with chemicals, Monsanto teaching the unsuspecting farmers how to increase their yields. No education on the dangers of these chemicals to their health, not to mention the adverse effect to those eating these crops. The same companies that introduced these toxic chemicals to farmers in Canada, back in the sixties, were now here, no chance.

Traveler was feeling like he wanted to participate at a different level in this dimensional shift that Mother Earth was deep into by this time. It was always the same response, he needed to transform himself, continue the search within and trust that Creator, through guides or higher Self, would send the information when needed.

There were many habits to break, many memories to let go off, take the ego out of its position of control, and maintain the health of the body but Traveler had a way to go before he could enter into that depth of his journey. Every soul will awaken in their own way and in their own moment, but there are easier ways if one is ready. In reality it is our responsibility to do this work at some point during numerous lifetime experiences here. It is freedom at the other end of this effort, similar to completing High School and then Summer break.

Each new day began in gratitude and in connection with Source or some energy that allowed a feeling of peace and calm before stepping out to greet the day. Traveler thought that he was a fairly patient person but the language barrier in Ecuador along with the different culture was bringing up frustration, something that he was not accustomed to. Creator had a plan, part of it was to take down the ego. Traveler was feeling the heat, people laughing at him because they couldn't understand a word that he was trying to speak in Spanish. He couldn't express himself as easily as he could back home, not even close, but in Father's perfection the language barrier became a blessing. Traveler quit looking to connect to the outside world, enjoy the walks but with very little communication, more just observing how he was reacting to things that passed in his day. It became a little different game. He didn't understand what people were saying, so he was seldom aware if they were having difficulties or what was affecting their lives. It was a bit like living in a cave but inside the city. The reality was, Traveler liked to be alone, it was there that the world made some sense.

Yes... being alone can be almost perfect for a while but in there, the odd time, self- doubt would rear its ugly head and the mind was off and running. Traveler, take a look at all the beauty here on Earth, the boat rides back on the St Lawrence River, Caribbean Cruise, dining in some fine Restaurants, you are missing the boat Johnny... Take inventory big fellow, you're alone, you are living with a mattress, one pot, one pan, yep you have got it all. There were moments where he had a choice to make, head back to Canada and return to the money-making game or stay the course. Traveler allowed the ego to take its swing, but he was in this search for truth and ready for the long haul.

On this so-called spiritual path, Traveler realized early on that he couldn't get on the phone and push for results, it wasn't like working in sales or business. The work that was required was to be non-evasive and done in silence.

Traveler knew that his family probably figured that he was in a slump. He has lost the will to get out there and make money come into his life and perhaps there may be some truth in that valuation, but the goal was only one. He needed to step out on faith each day, confidence in his Creator, in knowing that he was on the right path. This path does not allow for much deviation if that is truly what one wants; was he ready. Traveler always had faith that abundance would come back into his life, but what was the abundance going to be... Making more money might have eased the pain, but Traveler had had that for quite a few years, earning more each month then he had over any period of a year previously. Did it make him feel good? Yes... but it did not fill the emptiness inside, nor did it take any weight of his heart. Non- attachment becomes a little easier when one is just plain and simple fed up with the world as it is, nothing much has appeal. As the ancient Masters of the East have repeated, when the student is ready the teacher will appear...

Journey Home

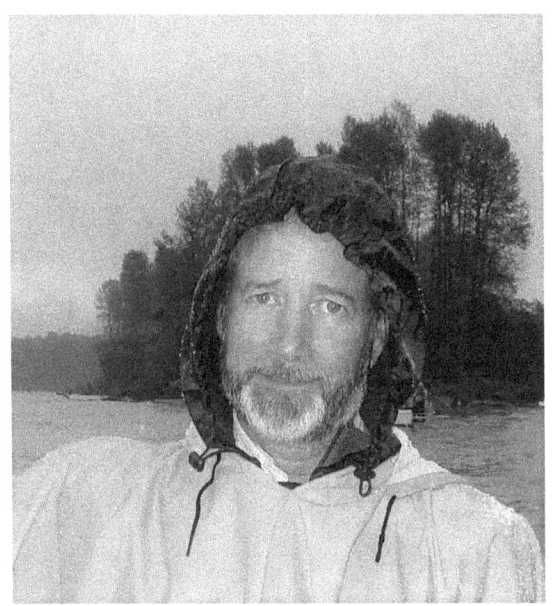

MAESTRO SAT GURU

Traveler had a reoccurring thought for quite a number of years, the thought that at some point he would like to spend time in another country with a Guru or a Spiritual Master. He wanted to meet someone who was Self-realized and that could guide him along the way. Not long after living in Cuenca the opportunity arose when he learned that Maestro Sat Guru was coming to teach for a weekend in April. There was only thing that he needed to know at that time was that this Maestro was a student of the same Guru, Sai Baba living in India, that Traveler was familiar with because other than that he didn't know much about the dedication that it takes to become a spiritual teacher.

Traveler had been aware of Sai Baba for almost 8 years, and he can only say that through his spiritual nurturing and love was he able to reach this point of devotion in his life. The highs and the lows, the seemingly successes and failures were an opportunity to develop equanimity and accept each moment as a gift. Traveler had definitely grown an affection for Sai although it was a slow process as the ego mind does not lay down easily and the world that most perceive at their conscious level, doesn't help to lessen the ego's grip. Traveler said that when Sai came into a dream it was as real as being here in this body. There were direct conversations with this being which always made Traveler feel special, as many devotees of his had wished for such an experience. One can show devotion through Jesus, Krishna, Buddha or even a tree if that is your choice. It matters not whether you have devotion to a form or to the formless as God exists in all, but ultimately you need to know that you are devoted to the one Source. There are many stages or steps on your journey and there is no wrong way, just try and be present as you take a fork in the road and then another and another. It only matters that you believe in some higher Intelligence that gives life and as we become more aware of the spiritual nature on this physical plane here on Earth, devotion is to that eternal fountain of Life, that mystery Spirit, to your Self.

The most significant part for Traveler at this time was the love that he felt swelling up in his heart, he hoped one day that he would be able to share that flow of love with all. He had a few miles to go yet... Sai's role in this world would come to light later on, but for now he was part of the learning and remembering for Traveler to experience.

As with all new ventures, Traveler attended the first introductory evening with Maestro with a little reservation and a fair bit of excitement. Maestro almost immediately began to share his experiences with this Sai Baba in India, which were over a period of almost ten years. This chat made Traveler feel more at ease. He soon became comfortable with the fact that Maestro's Vedic knowledge was in line with what Traveler was attempting to implement into his life. It would appear that Traveler was as apprehensive as a long-tailed cat in a room full of rocking chairs but he was at a point in his life where he did not want to take any wrong turns or be out of alignment with his spiritual journey, at least not if he could avoid them. Maestro was very much in tune with where Traveler was on his learning/remembering curve, and he was open to listening to Maestro's knowledge.

Maestro although felt the presence of God in his life at an early age, he began his spiritual journey in earnest at the age of nineteen. He had spent many years in India and also Thailand and was in the presence of a number of spiritual Masters whom he had become a disciple of or student of during his life thus far.

He fulfilled a yearning that he had felt for a number of years and that was to spend a year of his life in mediation, which he did. Each day for 20 hours he sat in meditation only coming out of the room for a hand full of nuts and raisins, before returning to meditate. The 4 hours left for sleep were often not required as the body was already rested. The mind finally lost its ability to a focus until it could not even recognize the surroundings in his meditation room. Finally, he reached a point of Self-realization witnessing the Oneness of creation and from a point in space viewed the Earth before returning to the senses of the body. He asked Bob Fickes, who was his teacher at that time, what now…the answer was to return to an active life here on Earth. Maestro says that one needs to gain Self-realization through the use of the body and mind while participating in life's experiences. It does not always require a grueling experience such as Maestro accomplished to reach the goal, each one has his or her own path or way.

Maestro's weekend seminar was held at a small Spa in the South end of the city. That morning Traveler went back to the house where Maestro and his wife Aum were guests thinking that the seminar was being held there, ah… still not catching on to all the Spanish words. As luck would have it, they were just leaving for the Seminar, and he was able to catch a ride with them. There were nine students in attendance the first morning including Traveler. Although much of Maestro's talks were given in Spanish, he would always bring Traveler up to speed in English and at break time they were able to have further discussions. It was the first time since leaving Canada that Traveler was able to participate in a spiritual talk, it was a good feeling.

Over the weekend Maestro shared many stories about his experiences along his own journey which is so important for other spiritual aspirants to hear. It was such a pleasure to be around like-minded people and feel at home. By the end of the weekend, they all had enough new techniques in hand to take home and put into practice in their lives.

Over the weekend session they learned two visualization techniques to be used with a one-word mantra and yantra, one of which was to kick start a rhythm in their body. On Sunday evening Traveler put the Dream meditation into practice before going to bed. This meditation technique is for clarity of dreams and also to open up energy channels, bringing in the Light. Traveler sat ready for quiet time and within the first minute there was an energy beam that was coming into his 3rd eye with quite some force until it finally pushed his upper body straight up and pulled his hands apart from their cupped position to being separate on top of his lap. The energy was so strong that it was making his eyes flutter rapidly while maintaining his body up. He was held in that position with this energy flow for 5 or 6 minutes and then it abruptly stopped, dropping his body onto his lap. Traveler thought, okay that should be enough for tonight and went to bed. He had had strong influxes of energy before in meditation but none with as much power as this one.

Before Maestro returned to Colombia, he had asked Traveler to attend his upcoming Seminar in Santandercito an area North of Bogota. With Maestro's kindness in offering food & lodging for Traveler during his stay, the decision was made to travel to Bogota in June. The anticipation of being in the presence of many like-minded souls was similar to waiting for Christmas morning to arrive when he was a child. Never doubt

Great Spirit's power and his love, if something is required in your life it will be provided, just trust that it is so…

After spending the evening with Rod and Pierrette in their home in Cumbaya, he boarded the plane in Quito and Traveler was on his way. He was greeted at the Airport in Bogota by Natalie, a member of his host family and Jorge a friend and a student of Maestro. Jorge said that their English was not very good but that they had big hearts, the latter certainly was true and became more and more evident as the weekend unfolded. Traveler felt at home immediately with these wonderful Colombian people.

The first night was spent with his host family, Arturo and Pilar along with their two children Natalie and Cesar. Natalie's English was quite good so with Traveler's limited Spanish they were able to share stories and experiences. Maestro has been a part of this family's life for many years throughout Natalie and Cesar's childhood.

Spiritual devotion is not something external for them, it is a way of life. One room in their home was dedicated as a place for meditation in the presence of photos of their teacher Maestro, along with the lineage of Spiritual teachers traced back to Babaji. Although no birthplace or name is known for Babaji he is said to have been on Earth since the time of Jesus the Christ. Paramhansa Yogananda mentions in his Autobiography that Babaji revived the science of Kriya Yoga.

Ecuador is beautiful and diverse, but Traveler was equally impressed with Colombia. As they travelled North, he saw that much of the valley was filled with Dairy Farms, bringing him memories of home. Colombia's infrastructure is similar to North America in many ways, but their cost of living is much lower. The bus soon arrived at their destination, a little behind schedule but breakfast was waiting for them along with the organizers for this event, ready to help get everybody settled into their rooms for the weekend.

The location was perfect for holding this spiritual gathering with Cabañas dotting the mountainside each connected with stone walkways. There was a babbling brook splashing over the stones which seem to draw one's attention to the beauty of the moment. Not all attendees were able to make it the first day, so Friday was a nice quiet start with Maestro beginning his teachings around Noon. Maestro was thoughtful enough to ask two of the attendees to translate the discourse for Traveler. Lia and Miriam did a wonderful job of keeping him in tune with the flow of information, a task not so easy, as they were eager to learn also.

Ignorance can be subtle as it maintains its' hold over humankind. As mentioned before, one's journey is unique, and each has a different path leading to the same unity and understanding. Up until this point in Traveler's spiritual life, most of his learning was through self-study and sharing of experiences with a few others that he had met along the way. Maestro came out the gate and into his search much different and at a younger age than Traveler. He was searching not only for the truth, but for teachers and spiritual Masters to guide him along. On Saturday Traveler began to understand the depth of this knowledge that Maestro was sharing and the sacredness in its presentation.

Mother Earth has been in existence for billions of years. There have been many teachers such as Krishna, Buddha, John the Baptist, and Jesus to name a few. These names are in reference to teachers and not intended to describe their lifetimes here or the significance that is held dear for each person. There have been a few significant teachers over the past five thousand years and many thousands of years before that. It is a pretty short time really, and their efforts were to try and shake humanity out of their sleep or awaken at least to the control that they were being influenced by.

Here we are today under the same influence of a few and even more effectively than it was a few hundred years ago. Today technology has given us more conveniences for many of us on Earth, but it has also made it easier for governments and individual greed, to control rather than assist their fellow human beings. One could look deeply into food additives, condiments, processed meats, consumption of meat raised in confinement and other products to see if there is a relation to the addictions that also keep consciousness in this 3D experience. Beware of the habits that seem so normal, everybody is doing it, must be right, right?

This moment in time space is two-fold as Mother Earth groans from the abuse of humankind (not so kind) and the destruction of nature on our planet, her life force that sustains all living things including humanity. Mankind is responsible for their own suffering, if we choose to be lead from day to day in ignorance then we cannot blame anyone else. It is about choices, our choice on how to live a healthier lifestyle and how we treat each other during our daily interactions. Can we forgive another and understand that they are functioning or experiencing life from their own perception, which is not the same as anyone else.

It is also a time of Light as many are beginning to awaken to their reality, their truth, the unity of creation and the potential for all within this great evolving adventure. This is the moment where so much light and energy are flowing into Gaia and our planet, this Grace is available to assist those ready to transcend this dimensional experience. It is not about leaving the body and going somewhere else, it is staying in this human instrument that can facilitate your journey home, your ascension path. Our planet's ongoing and upcoming global disasters will not be pleasant for many, yet there will be others less affected by these events. Preparation is key, not just with a few extra supplies on hand but your earnest effort to open up your connection to Source, through your heart.

Part of spiritual development requires maintenance of our bodies not only through good eating habits but exercise. Each day while Traveler was in the retreat in Colombia, instructors would guide attendees through a session of Tai Chi and Yoga coupled with breathing techniques to help bring more life sustaining prana into their bodies. Both of these exercises help to open up meridians and chakras which in part facilitate the flow of energy through their bodies. Quite often there is other healing required to open up blockages in the flow of Chi that may have been caused by accidents, trauma or negative energetic patterns from this lifetime or previous ones.

Traveler had read many times and heard from a few people about Gurus giving Darshan but once again Traveler was ignorant to exactly what it was. Maestro gave Darshan to the group 3 times over the weekend which had a different effect on each one of them. It is the teacher's focus on sending energy/love out through the heart center to those in a position or willing to receive it. This Love that poured forth from Maestro caused Traveler's heart to feel like it was filling his chest area, here was that pressure again, although he felt calm inside, his heart was aching. There are many reasons for the heart center to feel tight or blocked, lost love, emotional abuse from parents, teachers and the list goes on. It can be opened; one needs to be available for the moments that higher Self has ready to guide this transformation… There is no wrong way or right way, all is part of the search or experience.

There is an Egyptian legend that says at death our hearts are weighed on a golden scale by a black Jackal called Anubis. The heart is weighed against a feather and if the heart weighs more than a feather the soul returns to Earth for another lifetime. A child is born with this lightness of being, 100 percent in the moment with unconditional love, oh… how quickly the memories of the body and new programming takes hold of their experience. Traveler was not aware of this as he raised his own children.

On Sunday evening all attendees enjoyed sitting around a bonfire while roasting a few marshmallows. Traveler was sitting beside Maestro listening to him share a few stories of his journey and experiences with Sai Baba from India. He asked each of the self-realized people to come over one by one and share their story of self-realization. Each one shared the same sentiment that self-realization is not an experience, it is a reality for them, an absolute truth of their existence and each said that they see no difference between themselves and another or anything else that they see, all is Love there is nothing else. One by one they shared the moment of their self-realization and other than location all were the same. They cried and they laughed during that moment as they completely let go, allowing for the truth to reveal itself. They no longer felt as an individual but recognized that all is one with all of creation. The path towards the truth seemed a little clearer… Traveler was trying to understand this moment without judgment, it would take some time before the pieces of the puzzle were put in place.

Each and every day souls are awakening to something greater than themselves, a higher intelligence flowing in and around them. Life with all of Its potential and their access to this Greatness is truly within themselves. Individuals are becoming aware of their part in this game of life or adventure which is shared with our cosmic brothers and sisters. Each one in their own way and in their own time. Our human existence and experience in these instruments or bodies is truly a gift by the grace of our Creator. Of course, not all of the daily experiences are recorded by the soul, but the highlights are part of the character building taken from each lifetime. Being present in quiet time or meditation is the moment where answers to questions can be revealed, something that has eluded humanity during different moments of evolution on this planet earth.

As more souls awaken, during their journey toward the truth of their existence, their connection to Source continues to open. Many times, during this journey our friends change, and we are attracted to a different frequency, those with a different level of consciousness, more in alignment with our own. Yes, for sure the law of attraction is at play. Perhaps harmonization of humanity and all life forms on earth seems like a remote idea, but it is not. Each one of us is responsible for this shift in consciousness and it can only be accomplished by our individual effort, however small or great that is.

Traveler was reflecting on his journey to date, and it appeared now that there are a few spiritual check points along the way, where one is able to reference their progress. It is important to be open and ready to receive, letting go of all expectations. Maestro said that each seminar contains within it, information for all in attendance regardless of where they are on their journey. They receive the information that is relevant for their understanding and perception. It is a process to open and expand their hearts to a point where a person can finally begin to let go of their inhibitions and allow for their divine Self to shine through and reveal their truth.

One eventually goes beyond the desire for more of what the material world has to offer. Perhaps more accurately said is that one becomes absolutely fed up with it all, for a while anyways… The pendulum eventually begins to center to a point where it is possible to appreciate the grandness of sharing life on this planet. All experiences which one might perceive as good or bad can really be beneficial to the Soul's journey during their awakening.

There is a grand idea held by Source which sometimes does not make sense at our level of understanding. These polarities eventually cease to affect the mind so that our soul can just be in peace and calm which is its true nature. Our emotional body is truly a gift to this experience but in order to continue ascending to the higher levels of consciousness, it will be required of the individual to master the emotions.

As Traveler looked back life seemed like just a flash in time. There were many things that he had experienced during the Retreat and now it was a time of digesting and reflecting on this information. It was certain that the mind was the cause of most of the pain that life seemed to be dishing out, so the task at hand would be to try and quiet it. Where was it getting its power over Traveler's experience? Maestro said that realizing the Self was like a starting point on the journey, it was a pretty broad statement, but Traveler was determined to stay the course.

Traveler truly felt loneliness after returning from Colombia and perhaps a bit estranged. It is difficult to explain the experience that he had shared being around this group of spirit loving people. There was a feeling of love that emanated during those three days, just from being together. Yes, the old ego could quickly say, "Horse manure, get a life." This love or feeling is ever present throughout all that exists. It is ever patient, never wavering and just waiting for a Soul to be open enough to receive and to share.

What is it that stops a person from just enjoying the moment to the fullest, like a child discovering each and every moment as being new? Traveler was a few years away from really getting into the depth of these crippling energies that were still causing havoc in his life. One that perhaps is prevalent in our lives is doubt, it doesn't have any power until a person believes in it. Start believing in your self-doubt and it will soon anchor your life in this cesspool. Why not change over to living in confidence, a trust in the fact that Source will look after all that is required.

Traveler remembers a man from his hometown, he was called the Duke of Doubt. He was a good man, by the world's perception, worked three or four jobs in order to provide for his family. One of his part-time jobs was digging graves and another was holding the position of Fire Chief for the village. After every fire he would comment that, "Well we saved another foundation." Perhaps he was stuck in self-doubt, having difficulty in deciding to guide his fellow firemen.

A decision needs to be made decisively and we live with the consequences. If an error is made, then one has the opportunity to learn from it and use that experience for the next moment. As has been said by many Sages, it is best to not start the spiritual journey but if you do start, it is best that you stay with it and finish it.

While Traveler was in Colombia, Maestro had asked him to start initiated people in Ecuador if the need arose. Maestro had initiated Traveler on a few mantras and yantras, enough for the first level of Initiations. On the last night in Bogota, one of Maestro's assistants showed Traveler how to begin the Puja which was performed before each initiation. Traveler was a bit surprised when they started that evening, as this Lady began to clear the 4 directions of the room with a burning incense.

One morning in meditation just before Traveler made the trip to Bogota, he had had a profound experience. It began with a voice that said you are an ancient Soul here on earth, he was in a state of consciousness but leaving the dream state. It was like a contact from a higher Essence, was it God, he didn't know, but felt that it had some higher connection. It was comforting to hear this voice, sensed without a doubt that Traveler was just not this body here on Mother Earth but a being with much more depth to it. With this gentle wake-up call he got into a comfortable position for meditation and shortly into quiet time Traveler felt a hat like form on the crown of his head something that you'd see in India or Tibet. A bolt of energy came from above connecting to the point of this hat and rocked Traveler in vibration for quite a while. When this quiet time was over, Traveler stood up, like being in a trance but very conscious, lit an incense and began clearing the room, starting from the North than East, South and finally to the West. The form of an equal cross was made with the incense asking Creator to "Please remove all negative and dark energy from this place.", then bringing the incense back towards the right shoulder in 3 circling movements while repeating, "Allow only your Love and Light to be present." and then finally resting over the shoulder. There wasn't much chance of this being a coincidence. When one is open to receive… you will soon begin to know who you are.

MAESTRO IN ECUADOR

It was back to life in Cuenca for Traveler, teaching most days and trying to stay warm at night as Cuenca can be quite cool in the evenings especially when it rains. Traveler continued to take a few Spanish lessons and through that group of people he began to do a few initiations for Bija meditation. It was a time in his life where Traveler was feeling a deeper sense of being, perhaps now this was a purpose for his life. Oh… be careful, ego is always quick to assume its new role. It hung on to I am a farmer and after that past the ego continued, I was a farmer most of my life, blah blah blah. Traveler was unaware of this at that time, but soon he would wake up, or at least open his eyes.

It was late in 2007 when a decision had been made to bring Maestro back to Cuenca for another retreat and with the help of Tatiana arrangements were being put in place. It would be held in Baños de Cuenca just far enough out of the city to be a little more peaceful. Traveler and Tatiana were stepping out on faith as neither one of them had organized any type of event before. All fell into place, and everything was ready…

Life seldom remains without change for anyone, and this was no different for Maestro. He and his wife Aum made a mutual decision that it was time for a new chapter in life. Aum was returning to her homeland, and Maestro would remain in the United States, which had been his home sense he was a teenager.

By the time Maestro arrived in late December he was accompanied by Isis who would in time become his wife. Maestro had decided to arrive a few days earlier to help with the set-up and get settled into the Hosteria where the event would be hosted. Within the first day things started to fall in place with new contacts who had held spiritual events in Cuenca and were anxious to meet Maestro. Soon he was being interviewed on the local radio station and receiving recognition for his work. At this time, he had written a few books related to living in the heart, a great help to this Spanish speaking community.

The event was a success, perhaps not so much in the number of attendees but in the seed that was planted by his presence during those few days. There were students from Colombia who made the trip to be in front of Maestro once again, one of them was John who had endured a grueling bus ride from Bogota. Soon Maestro was being recognized for his healing techniques which he had acquired during his time in Asia, with one of the main influences coming from a Spiritual Healer in Thailand. Each evening she allowed her body to be an instrument for an ancient Healer coming in from another plain of existence, he was known as one who teaches the Masters. She healed thousands of people who lined up at her door from evening until mid-night each day.

Within a few days after that weekend Maestro decided to stay in Cuenca, set up a space for healing and began his Healing practice. Each week there were other small seminars being held to educate interested parties on meditation and the benefits that it can have on one's life. Maestro and Traveler became good friends along with Isis and shared many laughs, many moments of revelation.

As Traveler was still living lean, Maestro taught him without charge, initiated him in other levels of meditation, Arch Angel energies and all levels of Reiki. It was a beautiful time for Traveler, so blessed to be around this group of Souls continuing to open up to their eternal connection to Creator.

Soon there were small groups in Guayaquil and Quito, keeping Maestro busy. He and Isis stayed for a number of months before heading back to Florida for a while and then returned in September which would see them in Ecuador for almost another year. How blessed they all were to have a guide for their spiritual adventure, right here in their backyard.

It was truly a wonderful time being present and listening to other people´s experiences that they had experienced through meditation and as well see the changes in their daily life as they became more aware of the necessity for balance. Creator seemed to have it all laid out perfectly for Traveler, felt like he at last belonged here on earth.

Traveler's son Rory came to Ecuador early on in 2008 and spent some time with Maestro in Quito for a Puja and then for a hike up to the base camp of Cotopaxi, the white capped volcano. This was a special day; Traveler hadn't seen his son in almost two years, so they were anxious to get caught up. During the day there were a couple of Eagles floating over-head, could be past lifetimes as a Native Indian but Traveler always felt that anytime an Eagle joined the moment it was a good sign.

They drove up to almost 4500 meters above sea level and from that point they had to walk up to the base camp situated at the snow line. The group were not too far into their climb when they looked over-head to witness two huge Condors floating as if they were in slow motion. What a feeling to see these historic birds, definitely pulls one into the present moment. It was a difficult climb; each step brought a little lighter feeling in the head and shortness of breath. Rory could not figure out why he was not able to keep up with the ole man, but Traveler had been jogging steps in Cuenca at 2500 meters above sea level for a number of months and was more accustomed to the altitude. If it was not for the thought of hot chocolate and soup at the camp they might have bailed out and turned around. They eventually conquered the climb and enjoyed lunch as well as a short snowball fight.

The next morning Rory and Traveler were on a flight to Manta a small city on the coast of Ecuador. Within a couple of hours, they were checked into their hotel and suited up for the beach. It was a great day, switched the hot chocolate up for a few cold beers and put some good ole hometown humor into the afternoon.

They spent a few days travelling by bus down the coast, through the small towns and villages of Puerto Lopez, Olon and Montañita until they finally ended up back in Cuenca. They spent a couple of days in this beautiful city before they headed to the Amazon, East of Zamora. I was a long bus ride but well worth it. On their first night they stopped just before nightfall at a small Hosteria where the owners treated them to a feed of frog legs, jumbo shrimp, breaded chicken, patacones (pan fried plantain) and rice. There happened to be a small wedding at this Hosteria, so they were invited for cake later that evening. Bright and early the following morning they boarded an Inter-Provincial bus headed for the town of Yantzaza, not too far from the border of Peru.

Traveler and Rory had lunch and figured out the next leg of their journey. Before long, a small bus pulled into the village, it was time to take another ride for the next couple of hours until they hit the end of the road. With their backpacks in place the boys walked another twenty minutes or so and finally reached their destination, a Hosteria nestled in the jungle along the riverbank. Zamora river seemed to be passing through the middle of nowhere, just what they were looking for. Their host was waiting for them and within a short time supper was being served, fresh trout with all the trimmings. Traveler's student in Cuenca was a young Doctor who had finished his internship in this remote area. He said to Traveler in class one day, "This place is almost unknown." He was absolutely right.

Early the next morning after breakfast they were on a long river boat headed up stream against a fast-flowing river coming out of nowhere. It was like going up a corridor, the rock faces on both sides were 40 to 50 meters high, with waterfalls cascading down on every bend. National Geographic definitely came to mind. After almost an hour and a half they docked at a small Indian Village. Yes, without a doubt, Traveler and Rory were excited to experience this, but it turned out that the same boat now provided access to the outside world for these villagers, so there were a few Native Lads passed out from drinking too much beer and trago (Sugarcane liquor). It is here, like so many natural wonders where tourism can quickly take the innocence out of nature. They walked for another hour or so, good thing they had a guide.

There was a cave waiting for them with a fairly deep flow of water inside. They climbed into the first part, not so bad, the second cave required sliding through a narrow crevice and into the darkness. They rolled the pant legs up and in they went. Moving into this absolute darkness brought deafening screams from this cave, there were at least a hundred Oil Birds flying overhead, but they could not see them, at first glimpse it was thought that they were giant bats, but fortunately not to be. The birds made their vase shaped nests out of their droppings perfectly placed on small ledges high on the cave walls. Each nest was home to one or two chicks. When they started taking photos the flash would light up all the eyes that were whisking around. The Oil Birds are nocturnal fruit eaters, apparently the Natives use them for their oil, hence their name.

It was even a longer ride home as it had been raining heavy in some areas that they had to travel through, sometimes the bus would stop for an hour or two, waiting for the equipment to clear the mudslides. It was truly an adventure that Traveler and Rory enjoyed sharing together. They spent the remaining days in Cuenca and then it was time for Rory to head back to Canada.

It was time to return to teaching for Traveler, earn a little cash to keep fresh bread on the menu. During the past year he had made a couple of trips back to the coast, but this time into the mining areas. A friend from Canada was looking for black sand, Traveler said jokingly that there was lots of it on the beach. Al was referring to tailings from the gold mines.

After a few trips up the mountain in el Ranchero (Flat-bed truck with seats), Traveler finally made a couple of contacts and gathered up some samples to ship to Canada. It turned out that there were well over a million tons of tailings just in one area and because the mines were not too efficient, the black sand still contained between four and eight grams of gold per ton, along with silver and copper. It took some effort, but this venture eventually took on a life. Later in this story…

In May of 2008 Traveler accepted a teaching job in Olon on the coast, as a volunteer. He received three meals a day and had a small apartment above the school, short commute… In reality everyday was another day closer to the truth, many habits and memories have to be rooted out, but until one finds out the necessity of this, it is a slow process.

Teaching all grades of elementary school kids requires a fair bit of patience, Traveler has a lot more respect for Teachers now. Some days the little characters just wanted to play around, sometimes slipping out of the back of the class and into the playground. Most of the time they were anxious to learn. There were a couple of times patience slipped away and Traveler caught himself being angry with the kids. It only lasted a moment, but it was long enough to see the craziness of it. The ego is slippery, and it likes to keep control. During their first month the children learned how to sing the Gayatri Mantra, in Sanskrit, it was interesting to see the kids heading home with their parents while singing this ancient song.

On the final day when Traveler was ready to leave, the teaching staff had a surprise for him. They had organized a sendoff from the students who stood in a group outside the school and sang the Gayatri Mantra. This was a special moment as all of the students wanted a hug before they left for home. These young children quickly become extremely attached to a foreigner and the feeling was mutual.

His volunteer experience ended and Traveler returned to Cuenca. Once he was back in the city there was no real work in place as almost all schools were out for summer vacation. It was a rather quick decision but fortunately he was able to return to Canada for work. Rory was junior Superintendent on a Hotel-Condominium Complex in Vancouver, so he was able to bring Traveler in for a few months to complete deficiencies on the project. Ah… Creator always seems to have everything in place, sometimes not what a person was looking for but exactly what is required.

Traveler first landed in Houston where he had a nine hour lay-over. He had about forty dollars with him, this could last a week in Ecuador. Oh, my friend you are not in Ecuador anymore, the price of food in the Airport was a bit of a shock, but one must eat. He landed in Vancouver with six dollars in his pocket and looking forward to spending time in beautiful BC.

It was great being back together with Rory and as well his brother Hugh and his family who lived in Burnaby at the time.

Charlotte was living in Pemberton, only a three-hour drive to the North. It would be a great summer...

The next morning after Traveler's arrival, they were at the jobsite, got some paperwork out of the way, took a little walk around the building and then off for breakfast, wasn't so bad. It was a fairly easy job with really good pay, so Traveler was soon caught up with the money that he had to borrow to make the trip. Yes, still living lean.

About every second weekend, Traveler would take the bus up to Pemberton to visit Charlotte. This area is truly a paradise, a long valley between two rivers and up from the rivers ascend the Rockies. There were Eagles over-head and hardly a day went by without seeing a black Bear. Traveler enjoyed every minute with Charlotte, they really had not had much time together since she had finished College. She had become a certified Yoga instructor, so Traveler was able to add a few more exercises into his daily routine.

They rode bikes, canoed down the rivers which were still cool coming straight down from the Glaciers. Most days would be spent going for a walk into the village for a coffee and meet a few locals. Grizzly was a local Artist, an older gentleman with a white beard and long silver hair. He and Charlotte had become good friends and he was giving her lessons on sketching and painting. Grizzly had been in Tibet for part of his life living as a Monk but eventually life brought him back to Canada. Traveler looked forward to these trips to Pemberton, they had a lot of catching up to do...

Back in Vancouver Rory and Traveler were together almost every day, what a way to spend a Summer with your son. Yes... there were a number of evenings spent sipping Ale, something about cold Corona on a hot Summer's eve. Although it was a little twist from Traveler's life in Ecuador, he still tried to maintain a sense of his spiritual process. It required getting up at four thirty in the morning for quiet time, but he became accustomed to the early wake-up.

One evening he awoke with eyes closed to a bright light. He covered his eyes with his hands and closed the eyes a little tighter but the light from within just kept getting brighter, almost blinding. It would be the beginning of this light shining brightly from within. Meditation was a habit for sure, Traveler could not imagine a day without it. Traveler had an opportunity to practice a bit of Reiki while he was there, a wonderful experience for sure.

Maestro had taught Traveler a couple of Falun Dafa exercises while they were living in Cuenca which sparked his interest. He looked for a teacher in Vancouver and within a short period of time Traveler found out that a teacher was living in the next apartment building over from where Traveler and Rory were staying.

June and his wife Helen met Traveler at the Park in front of the apartment buildings one Saturday morning. They were a wonderful couple, soft spoken with a genuine sense of humility. June shared a short story about the history of Falun Dafa, which had seen these exercises held in secrecy perhaps for thousands of years as it was only passed down from Master to disciple. These ancient exercises were not meant for public knowledge. Helen and June fled China as did many others who were in fear for their lives. It was a difficult and dangerous time as the Chinese government were persecuting those who were practicing this ancient wisdom. It seems truly amazing how governments use their force to limit the freedom and individual rights of humanity. Master Li has been teaching Falun Dafa and its principals outside of China since the nineties.

These exercises are wonderful for aligning energy channels while helping to bring harmony and balance into one's life. June went through the exercises a couple of different times with

Traveler until he had them mastered. Some of the advanced exercises were quite intense but they managed to get through them together. Traveler continues to use these exercises today and has maintained contact with June.

The Summer was coming to an end, and it was almost time for Traveler to head back to Ecuador. It was the night before the last day at work and Traveler and Rory decided to go downstairs to the Restaurant that was located in their building. Their plan was to share a couple of beer, enjoy supper and call it a night. They completed supper but stayed for quite a while after, telling stories, laughing, and sipping away. It was late when they finally got into bed and neither of them overly coherent. It was about five o'clock the next morning when Traveler awoke, oh oh, time to go to work. He took a look at his watch, still on his wrist and the hands had stopped at 12:12. Traveler said to himself, "I hear you Father."

He took it as sign that it was time to get serious about the journey once again. This date December 2012 had been resonating in Traveler for a long time, since early 1998 after landing in Mexico where he had picked up a magazine that had a full article on the Mayan prediction about a major change coming up in the world. This date was in the forefront of his mind, wanting to prepare somehow. The watch was an expensive one, but he could never get it fixed even though he tried in several places in Canada and Ecuador, so finally he just left it with a street vendor in Ecuador. Maybe it was time not to be so connected to time.

The day had come for his return back to Ecuador, Rory and Traveler had breakfast at the Airport and then said their goodbyes. No doubt that it had been a wonderful Summer with Charlotte and Rory, better moments, impossible. It is still a time that all three cherish.

When Traveler got back to Cuenca, he moved into a new apartment along the banks of the Tomebamba River close to the center of the historical city. It was more like a studio, but it had big windows to let the sun in, two sundecks with palm trees overlooking the river and its endless walkways along it. Traveler set up a special area for a few spiritual Masters, a place for quiet time, all was good.

Before too long Traveler was giving Reiki treatments at a Health Center which was across the river and within walking distance. There was a fairly good flow of people looking for treatments and it was great experience for Traveler. Each person had a different experience, some profound and others were very peaceful. Traveler was beginning to think that perhaps this was his purpose but not to be.

In reality there is fair bit, no… a lot of effort required to work on purifying the mind/body. He still had a warehouse full of memories that needed to be cleared. This moment in time performing Reiki combined with Arch Angel energy was extremely rewarding for the patient and for Traveler but there was another plan in place.

By the end of September Maestro and Isis were back in Cuenca to live and set up their meditation events and Health Center. It was not long after their return that they were back into the rhythm of small seminars and group meditations a few nights a week. It was great for Traveler to be back in tune so to speak. Maestro was always willing to share his wisdom and assist Traveler in his spiritual journey wherever he could. He could not have asked for more than that.

It was around the beginning of October when Traveler received a call from Rory saying that he wanted to come to Ecuador. Rory was having a tough time trying to control his drinking habits, so he needed some help. Traveler told Rory to come on down, the timing was right as he could join in with

Maestro each week to help with the healing. The old saying, 'the apple does not fall far from the tree', holds a bit of truth but the memories of alcohol abuse are in the genes. The memories go back in both lineages of Rory's parents so at some point the problem has to be cleared, easier said than done and which generation is going to do it...

Once again Traveler and Rory were living together, there was an extra bed at the apartment and plenty of space. Before long Rory was being initiated in different levels of meditation, as well as receiving the initiations for Arch Angel Energy, all which could serve as a method for self-healing his addictions. It is amazing how Creator's plan always unfolds in perfection. It is usually easier to see the perfect plan looking back as we normally get caught up in the turmoil that we are living through. Eventually if one can stay on the journey of discovering their truth, they will come to have absolute trust in Creator's grand idea for Life, which we are a part of. Living in gratitude will bring you in alignment with this beauty and goodness.

Rory and Traveler made a few trips to the coast during those two and a half months or so, to enjoy the ocean breeze on the beach and yes, an afternoon of refreshments. There was a fairly good balance, at least from their point of view. Living life to its fullest and staying the path of learning during time spent with Maestro. In reality it is all Life experiencing life.

By Christmas time Rory was ready to head back to Canada as he had fallen in love with Nicole and wanted to surprise her by being home for the holidays. The New Year brought changes for Maestro and Isis, and they moved to Guayaquil to set up another Healing Center. More people were searching for Maestro's wisdom and meditation practices.

Traveler was heading North to the Colombian border, to encounter many lessons that almost totally drained him physically and mentally. He was not looking for these lessons, he was looking for gold. The experience that awaited him was far beyond his comprehension. How could Esmeraldas, the most beautiful province of Ecuador, hold so much corruption and risk to life? Nature and its beauty stood peacefully even though it was rampant with crime and murders every week. Most, if not all gold producing groups were being taxed by the Columbian FARC, another book could be easily written on their effect in this border area.

Through his contacts in the mines on the coast he decided to join Franklin on a small gold extraction project near the village of Borbón and not far from San Lorenzo. Rory and Traveler had made the trip in the Fall of 2008 and decided that it would be worth a try. Oh, my friends, darkness plays during the day in this place.

Traveler and Franklin lined up equipment to ship to the site along with supplies necessary to get started and within a short time they were heading North. The first couple of weeks were spent in Borbón which is situated along the river delta between Ecuador and Colombia. You could easily find the two Canadian Hotel guests as they were the only white folk in town. It seemed like a great place, at least for restaurant meals, as the coconut chicken was unbelievably delicious, at a price of less than three dollars.

Esmeraldas has quite a history and from that moment when a ship was stranded off the coast of Ecuador in 1533, it would be the first group of Afro-Ecuadorians to settle in this beautiful province. These first settlers had to battle with the Native Indians of this area in order to survive. By the time this fighting ended the original group suffered the loss of many lives. Slavery in Ecuador continued by different groups, including the Jesuit priests, up until 1852.

Their first couple of weeks were spent visiting the property near Selva Alegre, a small settlement far off the main road, close to an hour. Each day you could see the mules and horses loaded down with bunches of green plantain and bananas coming out of the bush or walking along the dirt road.

Almost everyone carries a machete, normally with an edge similar to a Samurai sword. Two men offered to cut a trail around the property line so Traveler and Franklin could see exactly where they could start excavating and set up Camp. They started in one corner near a small creek, it was like something out of a movie as they cut a swath almost three meters wide. Any saplings that were two inches or less in diameter were taken down in one swipe of the machete, there was seldom more than two swings at the same branch. Traveler was excited to be there and witness this raw strength but in another breath, he was wondering if he was nuts. This was a long way from home.

Although they secured the land and permission from the municipality, within days the federal government sent in the Ecuadorian military to enforce new laws. Part of their presence was because of the breach of existing mining laws by many groups, and the other being that this area was being plagued with extortion by the FARC. As this situation continued to unfold the decision was made to make a move to another area owned by a small group of Indigenous, more like a red-neck community who had title to over 1,000 hectares. This was one "forking" cross in the road that should have been well surveyed before taking a left and continuing on blindly. Bad to worse is putting it mildly.

Up until now it was still a bit like a tourist adventure with a contract or two, but the reality began to unfold when they hired a boom truck to move a large piece of equipment from Selva Alegre. Selva Alegre means "Happy Forest", ah my friend this place was anything but happy on this day, especially for Traveler. Mr. boom truck operator decided he could not get close enough to the machine to pick it up and despite Traveler's pleas in his limited Spanish it was to no avail.

As bad luck would have it, a logging Skidder was in the area and suggested he pull it closer to the road. Traveler was screaming by this time as he could see the inevitable destruction flashing by like a vision from hell. Franklin had his arms folded resting on his bulging belly almost all the time during this fiasco, that should have been Traveler's signal to head back to Cuenca. It seemed like an eternity before they finally loaded the smashed equipment onto the truck. It was now long after the sun had set and darkness was cause for another concern, so they needed to get a secure area to park the truck over-night. Nothing is left on the streets for the night, or it will disappear, without a trace.

Here is the spiritual part of this episode if one is trying to wake up. Traveler had never experienced such anger in all of these years of life here on Earth. He could not figure out where it was coming from, he had been so calm most of his life, what happened now. There were actually moments of, I would like to drag these animals (men) out of the vehicle and knock the living crap out of them. He could not even get satisfaction by screaming at them, not enough Spanish words to be effective.

Traveler had noticed one time while riding the bus on the coast that he was having thoughts that were not normal for him, so he figured it was like another grid of consciousness in that area. This might have been a tiny part of this situation with the equipment move, but the reality was Traveler would soon realize that there was a lot of suppressed memories that would need to be cleared out of his physical and emotional bodies. Purification or healing was way off in the distance, hardly even a word at this point.

Early the next day this smashed piece of equipment was moved to San Lorenzo. This small city is by far one of the most dangerous places in Ecuador, it would make Borbón look like a Sunday school.

They dropped the equipment off at the repair shop and it was agreed that it would be ready in a few days. Traveler and Franklin returned to Borbón to pick up their belongings and find a Hotel in San Lorenzo, which was also situated on this beautiful Delta. It has a wonderful history as the main Inland Port for Ecuador, from this small city cargo could be received by sea vessels and shipped to Quito by railroad and vice-a-versa.

This is the part where doubt begins to settle in about Franklin. He decided to take the bus back to Machala for a few days to visit the family while the machine was being fixed, fair enough. Frankie boy was to make arrangements for his part of the investment in this little project but with each new day there was always another story and little money. Franklin returned the following week when Traveler, and he made their way into the jungle to meet with the Awas. In reality they passed through one village of real Awas who were, for the most part living traditionally in the AWA Reserve. It was considered a blessing for the young woman to give birth, so most of them were mothers at the age of thirteen.

There was the Mira River to cross and on this day the water was too high to use the truck, so it was time to take of the shoes and get wet. Their group had to walk another hour before they reached the village. It was a long walk up and down the mountain but worth it for the beauty, as the Toucans flew beside the trail, small waterfalls were hidden behind dense foliage. Nature has a way of putting calm back into the moment.

When they were crossing through the gate into the second village there was a huge black Snake that crossed almost at their feet, it had 3 places where its back was moving at the same time, so it was long. Traveler asked Maestro by email shortly after, if that was a sign. It was moving right to left so it meant that there was a snake in the group, turns out they all were. There is a small river by the village, in some places it was more than four meters deep, but the water was so clear it was difficult to judge the depth.

By the time they came through the entrance the families of this village were all waiting, and as you can imagine, the thought of sharing some gold with this community would change their lives a bit. They were soon sitting in a couple of dug-out canoes heading down stream guided by the men with long poles pushing from one side to the other. There was only one woman in this group who really knew how to pan the gold. She used a gold pan made out of wood and could spin it like a top just at the right angle until the gold was settled in the bottom. All of the material that they were digging out the riverbanks contained a fair bit of gold. Each shovel full had enough visible gold to verify that for sure there was gold.

Within a couple of days Traveler, Franklin, and a couple of Elders from the village were in the lawyer's office to sign an agreement so that they could begin moving in the equipment. First thing the next day the pump, generator, mattresses for the workers and supplies to set up camp were loaded on the truck and on the way to the village. Franklin headed home one more time to line up (supposedly) the cash and all was good to go.

It is a long story, and it does not get any prettier. After a few weeks, the piece of equipment that had been smashed, was now repaired. On the day before Traveler was set to transport this machine to the village, he happened to be out early that morning driving in that part of San Lorenzo. He came upon a few guys loading Traveler's equipment unto a flatbed truck, apparently the Welder had sold the machine at a discount and skated out of town. It was after a long-heated discussion that the buyer actually put a contract out on the Welder, five hundred dollars to take his life, just like that. Traveler should have headed back to civilization at that point, but he was still thinking about gold…

After a few hours of discussions, calm returned to the situation and someone finally contacted the Welder by phone, and he agreed to give the money back. Traveler should have returned to Cuenca but the lessons to learn were here. In San Lorenzo during these months there were at least three or four fatal shootings per week. All of the merchants in this small city staged a demonstration one day, closing their stores to march the streets in hope for more police action. This saga went on for more than four months and in the end not enough gold to make it worthwhile.

One day near the end of this experience Traveler was walking back into the Awa village and as he reached the top of a small mountain he sat down on the ground, whopped, not from the walk but from all the events that he had lived through. After a while he sensed something looking at him, he soon caught the gaze of a large white Falcon with a band of black, like Zorro, covering his eyes and back behind his neck. He would move his head back and forth, side to side like he was trying to figure out what was wrong with Traveler. One cannot stay in that dog day state for long when nature comes to play or make light of a situation. Traveler thanked the bird and Creator for that moment and continued on with a little more zip in his step. He later found out that the true name of this bird is the "Laughing Falcon".

Before they could move all of their equipment out of the village to be sold, some of it had been stolen, might have been an inside job... Seems like everyone felt that they should have their share. Traveler had reached the point of explosion many times, and he halfheartedly question himself, what happened to love all – serve all. It was only anger, frustration, lack of trust, disappointment, and whatever other emotions that a human being could possibly experience.

On the day that Traveler was leaving this place for the last time, the FARC were moving in with hundreds of thousands of dollars in new equipment, washing money so to speak. Creator new that it was time to get out, just needed a little push in the right direction. Traveler had come from a culture where a handshake was enough, this place was beyond his comprehension.

Traveler's last night was an experience that was new to him. He awoke feeling that his body was lifting up from the bed, but it felt so heavy. It lasted for a minute or so, and then the body felt like it dropped back down again.

He caught the bus to Guayaquil the next day and planned to spend some time with Maestro and Isis. After his arrival he shared some of the stories with them. Maestro said that he had had a similar experience with the body lifting up, it is the soul wanting to leave, it feels that it cannot take any more of the experience. Traveler believed it… Maestro was quick to point out that Traveler's Aura was distorted, and all of his energy fields were out of balance. It took a couple of weeks after returning to Cuenca where Traveler finally felt whole once again. In that type of environment, one should clear the dark energies at least each day with a salt bath. Traveler wasn't quite aware of the damage that these energies can cause and the need to clear them on a regular basis.

There were many things that Traveler learned from that experience, all things in life are spiritually related somehow. The body-mind-spirit are here as one, although it is a little more intricate than that. Traveler was happy to be back in Cuenca, back into a rhythm more conducive to life. He now knew that these emotions such as anger were still there, how does one release these memories… It would take some time yet before those answers would come.

Traveler had been in regular contact with his partner in Canada while he was in San Lorenzo. It had taken a fair bit of effort to collect samples for the tailings project and on the other end Al was getting the analysis done as well as testing out the extraction process. After many months it looked like they had a viable venture, ready to put a plan in place.

By mid-year they had a new mining company incorporated in Ecuador complete with bank account, lawyer and accountant. Their lawyer is a friend of Traveler's, someone that he could trust. Ecuador has a lot of beauty, but corruption is a reality. A signed contract with witnesses has no value unless it is signed in front of a Notary.

Al was busy looking for a few business partners to provide the required capital to put their plan in place. It was at this time Traveler moved to Machala to be closer to the mines, which are all within 1 to 2 hours of this coastal City. When Traveler arrived in Ecuador he came with 3 bags, now he needed a small pickup truck to make the move… living in high cotton. He found an Apartment in Puerto Bolivar on the seaside and before long he was settled in.

The next few months were focused on contacting mines to see if they were willing to sell their tailings and at what price. The location for the company's plant would need a good supply of water and road access to the storage ponds, not always possible as many are built on the side of the mountain. It was back and forth to Cuenca a number of times to sign more documents for the company. Al and Traveler were trying to get a tentative agreement in place with no cash in hand, so it took a little skating.

By the end of Summer there was another small injection of capital and now the company was beginning to come to life. Traveler had yet to meet a woman in Ecuador that he was interested in for a relationship. He had asked Creator for many years, if it was meant to be, that this partner would be someone who was more spiritually awake than Traveler was. By this time, he had kind of put the idea out of his head. This is where the story turns to love and a whole new definition to this word. If there was ever a fork in the road that changed his world, this would be the one.

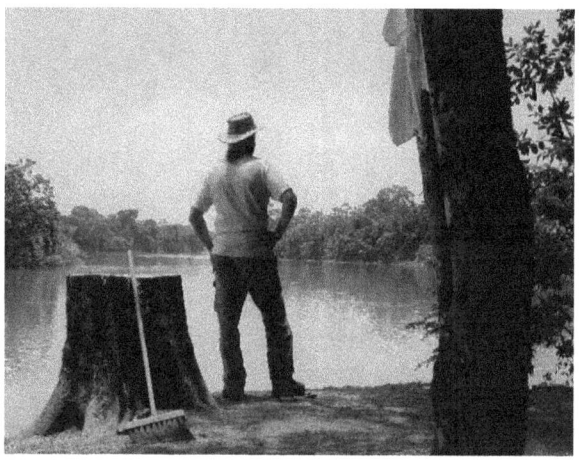

LOVE CHANGES ALL

It is a moment of gratitude for Tata Inti/Ra and Pachamama/Mahii as they give life to this experience here on Earth. Without Father Sun and Mother Earth our play of existing here on this planet would not be possible. Traveler remembers his moments as a young lad sitting on a branch of the big Maple tree or laying in the tall grass, feeling the warmth of the sun and the caress of the Summer breeze. It seems easier to understand a child enjoying this healing experience, without guidance or the need for details, just innocently connecting.

A person can become confused as the programming from the outside world continues pulling them out of their connection to Source. As powerful as Tata Inti and Pachamama are, they are eternally our brother and sister... Over the next few years Traveler would begin to understand the significance of ceremony and its importance as humankind consciously evolves through a better understanding of Self. As more of your daily thoughts focus on spirit (heart center and breath) and less attention on the physical, then the journey within takes on a life of its own. It is easy to get distracted in our daily lives but little by little our focus can be redirected to our connection with Source. Daily life still continues but as a much richer and peaceful experience.

Traveler's move to the coast would bring many significant changes into his life experience in Ecuador. He would experience dark energies firsthand and begin to understand how they move about in this dimension and within the astral plane. Business would once again try and consume him; decisions are made staying true to himself and his Self-discovery.

Late one September afternoon Traveler met a woman who would change his perception about love, passion, compassion etc. and life itself. Traveler knew that love seem to have different facets to it, love for a son or daughter is a love that goes beyond reasoning, it is a love that protects their life at all costs. Love for an animal seems to be more accepting of life and death, not so concerned about the short time that they are with us. This aforementioned non-attachment for animals was probably engrained in Traveler's memory as a child. During the age from nine years old to fourteen the family seem to lose a dog every year as they would be hit by a car on the road in front of their home. After crying uncontrollably for the death of the first three he finally accepted the fact that one day his pet could be put to rest. This never changed his feelings for a pet, but it took away much of the attachment.

It is the wisdom of our Creator that keeps the ever-changing future hidden from most of us or at least until we are conscious enough to know what to do with it. If Traveler knew what was about to happen in his life, he would not have been able to sleep until the day finally came. Well, it came to him in the most unexpecting moment.

When Traveler saw this goddess sitting alone and felt her unsettledness, he decided to write a note for her on a napkin as his Spanish was still not up to par. He wrote, (Cuando tu tiene estres en su la vida es necesario por/para meditacion), translating to (if you have stress in your life, you could try meditating). For sure she wasn't expecting this note and looked at Traveler at least with inquisitiveness.

From that day forward they have shared their life experiences together, in love and in a love that has no strings attached. Traveler had a feeling in his heart that he couldn't quite put a handle on, it was hurtful, joyful, wanting to protect, compassionate and persistent. He tried to shake it off, this feeling could not be real whatever it is, but it was powerful and yet wonderful.

Each day their love became more rooted, it could not possibly become any stronger. It was like they had been together for a long, long, time. Traveler had his small altar set up for meditation in his new apartment, and Rishi had questions. She was familiar with Krishna but not Babaji or any of the other spiritual masters. She shared stories of her time spent with the Hare Krishna group in Quito and how wonderful it was to be in that environment. Yes, Traveler had his pocket translator burning up batteries. Rishi had asked the Maestro for this Krishna group if she could learn how to meditate but he said that it was only for the more senior members. Interesting how teachings get twisted around when ye ole human being (ego) gets in control.

Traveler and Rishi decided to do their first Puja ceremony on September 22, 2009. The Puja is sung in Sanskrit and can be quite powerful. This tradition was passed down from Babaji, an immortal being who has been on earth in the same body for over 2000 years. The Puja is used to invite the presence of the masters as well as great beings such as Vishnu and Brahma. It is an offering in gratitude for their assistance in bringing those present into the light, which dwells within the body.

The body contains memories as well as beliefs, and for some, dark energy that can cause interference to their connection, so one's true nature is hidden. The first step perhaps is to know that fact and then begin to clear away this interference and become like a child once again or become empty, Jesus and Buddha had left similar messages, as well as many teachers.

Traveler and Rishi placed fresh flowers by the altar as well as water, rice, fresh fruits, camphor, three incense and three candles. Incense was lit, the four directions were cleared, Traveler sang the Puja and then they sat down to meditate. Rishi was still deep into quiet time when Traveler opened his eyes, so he waited until she finished her experience. Traveler asked Rishi to share the experience of her first meditation. As she began to tell the story, it was like Traveler had received confirmation that there is truth in the somewhat mystical stories, especially those that he had read in the Mahabharata.

They both had tears welling up in their eyes as ancient mysteries became more lifelike that day. Rishi was in another time space, a wooded area where tall trees were decorated with vines full of flowers of every color of the rainbow. She was dancing with Lakshmi, Sarasvati and Krishna, almost floating over the grass tinted with a hue of blue. There were hundreds of celestial beings with decorations in their hair softly twirling in dance, in celebration, to and fro within this sacred forest. Celestial music filling their hearts, existence in their very being. Traveler was in gratitude for that moment and to Rishi for sharing her personal experience.

It was only the beginning, the door to the worlds beyond were now open for Rishi and each day would bring another reunion with life beyond this dimension, beyond comprehension. Traveler had completed reading almost 12 books of Mahabharata and each of Rishi's experience was like a moment going back in time, bringing these characters, these celestial beings to life. They are our brothers and sisters who are overflowing with eternal patience waiting for the moment(s) of awakening. Each shift in consciousness bringing with it a change in knowing and understanding.

There were many Pujas over the next month and a half for initiations in different mantra/yantras for Rishi to make use of. It was a magical time for Traveler and Rishi as well for her son Victor who joined in on a few meditation initiations. There were ceremonies on the beach, close to the apartment as well on an Island just a short boat ride from the Port. Every day was a celebration as they shared their lives together.

By the beginning of November, they had decided to look for a bigger apartment where they could live together and soon after they moved into a place in Machala close to the city's center. This apartment was on the ground level of big house, with the owner living on the second level. All was well, lots of space with 3 bedrooms, 2 bathrooms, living room, dining room and kitchen. Traveler and Rishi set up a couple of rooms, one for massage therapy and one for reiki and energy work. Traveler was still active with the mining company, but it still required more capital to put their plan in place.

Around the third week of November, it was becoming quite apparent that this place had a number of dense energies living there. Traveler had only experienced this type of energy once before; it was while on vacation in Nova Scotia. He was staying in an old home that had been converted into a Bed & Breakfast. He got up early for quiet time in the morning and shortly after he sat down, he could feel the energy crossing through his body. Traveler was a bit startled, but he called upon Creator and Jesus to protect him and almost immediately the energy disappeared or at least stopped its activity. This new apartment had a much bigger presence of this activity.

Traveler is sensitive to the energies and physically feels their movement, Rishi on the other hand sees them. She has been able to see them since she was a child, including duendies or gnomes.

Every night was like a horror movie, Victor was sleeping with the light on, trying to keep them at bay as he also is able to see them. Each night Traveler would call upon Arch Angel Michael for his protection and fill their bodies with this fire energy before going to sleep. Many nights after midnight the energies would start crossing through their bodies and the main bathroom would have a strong odor of urine almost like a boar (male pig). Traveler and Rishi could handle the movement, although it kind of put the nerves on edge once in a while, like a good scare, a really good scare.

They were doing herbal baths to clean their bodies of this heavy energy as well as using salt baths or showers. It was to no avail and eventually these energies found a weak point or point of fear in Rishi, this would become like a pathway for them. They didn't know what was happening as it is something that changes day by day and is very subtle.

Each day Rishi was having a more difficult time keeping her eyes open and would be going to lay down throughout most of the day, and usually in their bedroom. It got to a point where some days she would be in a dream state consciously trying to get away from the characters in this dream but could not. She would open her eyes and see the bedroom upside down and close her eyes again trying to refocus. It was wearing them both down until finally one morning Traveler had a chat with Rishi.

She had been talking about going to another part of Ecuador to be alone for a while, needed some closure to a part of her life. Traveler was not sure if she was wanting time away from their relationship or if there was a problem. He wanted to reiterate his sentiments to Rishi once again as he had done during their first few weeks which was to say, you are free. Their relationship would be built on absolute freedom to live as an individual but share their life experience as one and any time their feelings changed for each other it would be better to move on. Traveler was wondering, how could this love for each other, take a turn.

It was over breakfast that Traveler began to piece together some of the stories about Rishi's family and thought maybe it was there that a solution could be found. Her mother was known for her gifts in healing others. Rishi's grandmother and ancestors were from the coastal indigenous tribe in Ecuador. Her grandfather's lineage was originally from Africa. Rishi's grandparents on her father's side were mystical to say the least, her grandmother was a healer who was well known in Esmeraldas. They had information which was passed down through generations which could be perceived as witchery or as healing remedies, depends on who is using it. For sure it needed to be used correctly and as close as possible to the instructions indicated.

Traveler began to ask Rishi about her grandmother's work and if she remembered the methods for clearing energies. It took a while but finally the information started to flow to her and soon they had it written down. Traveler stuck the paper in his pocket, and they were off to the market to buy fruits and vegetables. When it was time to come back, Traveler asked Rishi where they could buy the supplies needed for cleansing, she didn't think that he was serious about doing the treatment but in reality, she was not in a good state of mind.

In Machala there are quite a few ladies that sell dry herbs especially for cleansing energies, normally for baths not necessarily for the use that Traveler had in mind. It is close to some of the Shaman work but a little more in depth. They bought some red and yellow ribbon and small bottle of pure liquor which was sold in the market. It was back home to begin. The treatment had to be done over a three-day period with each treatment starting at the same time on each day. There was a ribbon test to see what the severity of this attack was, which could be mild or close to death. Rishi was definitely in the danger zone. If the treatment is not successful it has to be repeated the following three days.

It was an interesting three days as the astral energy was not happy with the ongoing treatment. On the 3rd day another ribbon test was completed which indicated that the treatment was successful. Rishi felt alive again and both she and Traveler were now more aware of these astral beings caught between dimensions. This house was a portal for these beings so it would have been quite a challenge to clear them out completely.

By the end of February, they were ready to move to a quieter place up in the mountains in a small village called Casacay. When Rishi and Traveler had informed the owner that they would be leaving Machala, she was disappointed but not surprised. She said that there was a Physician and his wife living there before and after three months in this house they ended their marriage and moved out, as well the couple before them had the same results.

Fear is one of the doorways for these energies to enter another body, shame, guilt, feeling of not good enough are also another opportunity. These dark energies seem to be more prevalent in Ecuador, perhaps because Traveler had never witnessed anything like it before in Canada. In reality these dark heavy energies are everywhere, the world is not exactly as it appears to the naked eye. This experience in Machala was just the beginning, as one gets closer to the Light a grander truth is revealed. It's like when you enter a dark room and don't see anything until you flick on the light.

It was now time for the mining company to move forward, full steam ahead. There were many things to look after but the first item on the list was to purchase a vehicle which was a 1994 Land Cruiser. This vehicle is definitely built for the mountain roads and would serve them well for the next few years. Casacay is a great place to live, where the people maintain a simple life and always willing to help out where possible. It became a welcomed refuge for Traveler and Rishi after long days of travelling the roads of Southern Ecuador. The next couple of years would see many changes in their perception of life and how the company was unfolding.

By April Traveler was in California meeting with experts in the field of gold recovery and manufacturers of this specialty equipment. From there it was on to Canada to meet with Al and another business partner. It was also a chance to stay with Rory and Nicole for a few days and a quick trip up to Pemberton to visit Charlotte and her new daughter Autumn. Traveler was excited to meet his grand-daughter, first one in the family. It was always a special time for Traveler to be with family even it was just for a short time.

When Traveler returned to Ecuador it was back to the mines, collecting more samples to be shipped to Canada, California and South Africa. Al was trying to find the best equipment for the new plant, so testing had to be done by each manufacturer. By June Traveler was landing in Johannesburg to spend some time with the manufacturer and go over results of their assays. Time after time the analysis were more than good so they arranged for final payment of the equipment. Traveler spent over a week with Johan, the owner of the manufacturing facility. His ancestors arrived from Belgium over 200 years before, so Johan had a good history of South Africa and the changes that it had gone through especially after Nelson Mandela took over as President. One never really knows the story until he is face to face with it, the world media is geared towards deception many times. While Traveler was there, Johan was preparing for the next step of gifting his company to the government, within the following couple of years (by law) he would sign over 50% to them. There's room for argument on both sides, bottom line, South Africa is a tough little country with a similar level of corruption as Ecuador.

Johan stands a solid 2 meters in height and tips the scales at 350lbs or so. He was a University Rugby player and tough as nails. He had been in the Boer War, so he was accustomed to the site of death. He was like another Jim as he had an endless supply of stories, only difference was the content. Definitely he had a different outlook on his life and that of others.

He shared an experience about a time when he was returning to Johannesburg from the Congo possibly through Tanzania where he had to catch another flight, if he missed it that meant a twenty four hour lay-over. He arrived on time, but they had filled the flight, so he was about to lose his seat. Johan made his presence known with a few choice words and before long two airport security men with pistols pulled arrived beside him. They suggested that he quiet down and proceeded to escort Johan to the Chief's office. Johan pleaded his case to this man, the Chief of Security only smiled as he continued to repeat that Johan needed to calm down. After Johan was finally quiet the Chief said that we have a system we follow here and that is all. Johan caught on quickly and said to the Chief, "And how much does the system cost today?" Johan paid the fee and soon the guards were carrying his luggage directly onto the plane. Remember the plane was full… There was a man smartly dressed in a white suit and tie sitting comfortably in the front row, lots of leg room calmly reading the newspaper. These guards tapped him on the shoulder and said that he needed to report to the Chief's office. As the man walked down the stairs complaining to the guards, one of them threw his luggage out onto the tarmac. Johan miraculously had his seat once again and surely the other man was now being enlightened about the system.

Traveler experienced the bitterness there on both sides, the Africans feeling cheated and manipulated, no doubt about that but now how could they swing the pendulum of change. All of humanity has been under manipulation for thousands and thousands of years. Misinformation, fear tactics, confusion, keep mankind scurrying for security. There is no security and even less today with electronic money, it can be wiped out with the stroke of a key. Where then does security lie, only with Source. It is there that one can rest, maybe just for a moment until their knowingness and understanding grows. Overtime these periods of being connected become more peaceful, more of a reality.

Traveler returned back to Ecuador anxious to be together with Rishi once again. Chatting long distance by phone coupled with the language barrier was a bit trying, but Traveler was always happy to hear her voice. Traveler brought quite a number of amethyst stones back with him so that they could use them to build an energy field.

This energetic field can be set up anywhere. The crystals are placed in a square position exactly 3.14 meters apart (on the floor or wherever the field is required) and then another crystal is placed in the center of the square, two meters above the floor or above the level of the other 4 stones. This pyramid is wonderful for balancing energies and can be set-up around the bed or office, etc. One of the simplest ways to test for accuracy on the placement of the stones is to have someone stand outside the pyramid with their hands interlocked behind their back, another person presses down on the hands and usually the person will begin to fall backwards as they are not grounded. Have them enter the Pyramid space and repeat the exercise, if all is good it will be difficult to move them of balance.

Traveler and Rishi continued their healing work on each other, both had old emotional memory issues to clear as well as deep tissue work to be done physically. They were able to use many of the techniques that Traveler had learned from Wen Shu as well as through massage therapy which Rishi had learned. There was a lot of healing, and memories to be released so they continued this work as time permitted.

The company was demanding most of their time now as there were contracts to secure, housing arrangements for the workers as well as other equipment purchases to be made throughout Ecuador. This little country can be a bit of a culture shock when one decides to live here, but you can multiply that by 10 when it comes time to register a company. When you have a corrupt culture, statistically reported rating for Ecuador was in the top ten, there is little trust. Appointments get cancelled or there are late arrivals to scheduled meetings. What is agreed upon today has no bearing on tomorrow's talks. Their road system at that time was a disaster, one could not travel at night without risking their life, as unsuspecting potholes and speed bumps in the middle of nowhere laid waiting to take your vehicle into flight.

Traveler and Rishi always had a small over-night bag with them as it was often the case, they would have to spend a night in a hotel, no five-star ratings in these small mountain villages… Their quiet healing time and energy work was slipping away. If there was a spare day, they would head to the closest mountain stream for a picnic and try to connect with Mother Earth once again. Those were wonderful moments for them as well as for Victor who normally went along. Rishi could always sense other beings that were close to them, sometimes bringing a message and other times, just being present. It always made the day a little more interesting and made them feel like they were still on their spiritual path.

It was about here where the spiritual work required a little more depth, as the egos needed to be addressed and habits cleared. Traveler thought that he was quiet, but he confused that for being humble and that his ego was more related to egotistic, so he thought, "We're good to go." During that time, a couple of months had passed, and it seemed like all was going well, things were progressing with the company and their life appeared to be normal. Traveler whined every day about the amount of driving and the rough roads but in reality, he liked the grind made him feel like he was back in the saddle again. As his daughter said to him one time, "Maybe you have no business being in business."

Rishi became a little distant some days, especially in the evening after they returned home to their apartment. They were long days on rough roads, so Traveler thought that that was part of it. Asking if you are alright all the time does not help. Rishi was trying to figure if what she was feeling was correct or not. Language was still a bit of a barrier as well as the Cultural differences, but their love and deep affection for each other remained strong.

Finally, late one afternoon Traveler asked Rishi again if everything was alright. Oh… that swung the doors open for that conversation, where someone usually walks away in the heat of the discussion. Traveler might not have caught all of the Spanish words, just as well, but there were parts in there about his ego, his controlling nature and that she felt smothered, like an invalid. Traveler, so he thought, just wanted to look after her be close to her. He was eternally grateful for her assistance in communicating with their contacts, without her it would have been difficult to say the least and he believed that they were enjoying this life experience.

It was a little bit of back and forth in Spanish and somewhere in there the thought arose, "how could this happen in their relationship." Traveler was not awake yet… Usually when the conversation gets a little heated, and no headway appears to be forth coming, that is a good sign to become quiet and slowly walk away, not to be. Rishi was a little, a lot more in tune with the need to go deep inside their hearts to see the reasons behind her feelings and Traveler's as well. Traveler had never reached that point of discomfort without exploding in some fashion, usually anger or laughter. He was in this instance, aware that he had to overcome the fear of talking it out until they were at a point of really listening to each other and more importantly, was that he was hearing and understanding what Rishi was trying to express in that moment.

It took several uncomfortable minutes of Traveler listening intently, before his body and mind began to reach a state of calm as the fear or this energy that had surfaced, slowly melted away. Once that point was reached it was much easier to be transparent with each other and begin to let go of their concerns that were causing tension in their relationship. It would take at least a couple of more years before this ego was dissolved enough to begin reaching its natural state or function.

This moment had been crucial in their relationship, if they were not willing to go beyond discomfort then this tension would have arisen again but with much more power. Control was joined at the hip with his ego, so both were a problem that needed to be addressed. Rishi is a far better cook than Traveler, she can bring flavor in from the heavens, literally. When they were not eating at some roadside restaurant Traveler would cook a meal at home, sure Rishi could cut a vegetable or two, but he was at the helm. Traveler confused that control aspect as being a good husband.

Traveler forgot the fact that Rishi had been removed from her home at the young age of twelve and had to look after herself from that point forward. She had raised her son and lived independently in a country that does not offer much support. Rishi had survived homelessness and weeks without food during the early years, a life experience that Traveler could not even imagine. Rishi finally was able to participate fully in the kitchen after a couple of years and Traveler was more than happy to step aside and enjoy her creations.

They both had issues to clear, Rishi had been in a tough relationship for almost five years, so she was still a bit apprehensive. Traveler was still trying to figure out what all had transpired during his first marriage. Nobody wants to talk it over, just shrug it off, grab another beer and hope that it goes away. That attitude can function until both husband and wife learn to avoid each other and perhaps staying together more as a comfortable habit. There is commonly a feeling that one partner or both, feel that there is something wrong with me, it is my fault. Some relationships are together for the wrong reasons and the only way to truly find out is to communicate and be truthful to each other. If there is any kind of tension being felt by one partner, then it needs to be addressed. Tension is a frequency than can cause cell damage to your body/mind and ultimately to your health, so better to talk it over.

The ego/mind is on autopilot, never letting go of its position until each individual takes control of their own life experience. The ego is attached to its sense of power, to its possessions, material or perceived. It will thrive on being wealthy or living in poverty, it does not judge itself it only wants to remain intact and exist. Artificial Intelligence with its technical advances in the last fifty years would be a good comparative to our ego.

Fear can be used to manipulate humanity into a dependency on the world around them. There is a dependency on being employed to cover at least the basics needs and the list goes on. This topic could expand into another book, but we are all living in our own individual world, that mind space where we are functioning from each moment. It is in that space where the choices are made, or the individual allows the outside influences to direct their life decisions. Yes, it will be chaotic in that mind space if the influence is coming from outside forces such as advertising, restrictions, opinions, luxury, poverty, inhumanity, insanity, truth, half-truth, fiction, religious beliefs, right and wrong, moral decisions, sacrifice to survive, no hope in sight and no end to the cause and effect. It really does not matter who said this, but the parable has relevance, "I AM the Way." If we are looking for a way out of the chaotic, then the Way is your journey within. It is removing and clearing the clutter of our lives, connecting to that Peace that is our true nature, no search required. IT awaits you all the while, giving Life. As the voice said, "I am the first breath and the last." So, there is a good chance that IT is everything in between.

As the story goes with the Yogi and his disciples, he went outside and sat in a pile of crap, could have been from cows or horses but either one would suffice. He sat there and threw a bit of it around and said as much crap as you see here, there is many more times this amount to clear out of your body and mind... It would take a couple of more years before Traveler finally took the shovel out and began to remove this pile from within. It is not pretty work, never is, but there is no magic pill or potion. In reality the experience is too precious to skip over it, it is through the purification that one finally begins to know thy Self. It is through this experience that a true understanding of life's purpose comes, that is the beginning of freedom, being at peace with yourself and have compassion for others on their journey home.

By late 2010 the company was in full stride, one major contract was signed at the Notary's office in Cuenca which brought true value to the venture. This contract was worth over ten million and their mining company was set to realize at least four to five million in profit, the time of high cotton was coming. Traveler and Rishi continued on with equipment and vehicle purchases. A Company Bodega (Storage Yard) was built along with a small house for the guard to live in. They made a couple of trips to Peru to source out a Refinery and to look at the possibility of setting up a Peruvian company to facilitate payments for their concentration (gold, silver and copper). They made a trip to Cajamarca and got a first-hand look at how big the gold mining operations are in Peru and just how strict their security is. They managed to get a couple of good contacts, one that brought them to Lima where they met Max, a businessman and a University Professor for all issues related to mining. All seem to be falling in place.

Traveler and Rishi were still growing in their experiences with dense energies, once again these energies were domiciled in two other houses that had been rented for the company. Over the next couple of years a few other people required help to clear these entities out of their life. By now Rishi was being guided from within, usually a giant white Serpent would appear in her inner-vision and give her a forward look at what treatment needed to be done and where. It became clear to them that all exists in balance and harmony and as they were active in this role of clearing it needed to be done in a peaceful manner sending the dark energies back to where they originated from, all needs to be done from a neutral point of love. It is difficult to imagine but some of these entities have been given this work, so it is not just a matter of sending them away without cause. Split personality might be a good example of what actually is going on with a person who might need assistance. In this case it is perhaps more difficult for a family member or friend to understand the situation.

It was still while they were living in Casacay that Traveler heard the voice once again during quiet time early one morning. They were simple words but far reaching. The inner voice said, "Do not be confused by any man." At first Traveler thought about the businesspeople that he was dealing with, he was cautious as he had seen many of them with good intentions, but no rationale to their ideas. Many of them were just manipulating for their own gain, which is the dog-eat-dog world, perhaps appearing more prevalent in South America, but in other parts of the world it can be the same just with a little more polish.

With a deeper look Traveler could see that the message was perhaps more towards the spiritual side of life. In these times of great change on Mother Earth there is a more concentrated battle for light, those souls using their liberty to ascend and those dark forces needing the light to carry on with their plan. What does that mean for the souls that are seeking the truth of existence and their part in it? One needs to be aware of the darkness, many of those who are functioning in an influential position in this world have a higher level of consciousness. This understanding at a higher level is often used to manipulate the masses. It is unfortunate that this has happened because there is more than enough provided for all life forms on our planet, including humanity. Once again, we are responsible for the change, waking up and making the changes in our own mind space, our individual world that effects Our world.

There are many on our planet today appearing as gurus, spiritual teachers, holy ones, masters, avatars etc., who are knowingly manipulating their followers for personal gain, some of our world leaders could be included in this group. This is not really about calling anyone out of the crowd, we all live our life from our point of understanding or perception. No one on earth can rest in a decision to stop their journey home, we are all learning and remembering our way back to Source. Harmony with our brothers and sisters is a difficult choice, so many of us feel that our way is the only way, we have to rethink that if we genuinely want to evolve as a human race.

There are many teachers of the truth or at least of their truth on Earth at this moment, who are consciously living in the moment. They are here to assist in humankind's ascension towards the Light, perhaps publicly or quietly but in their own way participating in raising humanity into a conscious level of harmonization. Be open to apply what resonates well with your being and know that as one continually becomes more aware, your understanding of your truth will unfold. One must be constantly looking within for the answers, listening to their inner guidance. The answers may come as confirmation outside of yourself such as information held within a book or from an Internet source, but one must move forward on feelings from the heart not from the mind. Traveler would eventually encounter the meaning of center or heart and how to begin to live from there but for now he was still ego bound to the business world trying to balance the spirit with material. He would remain out of balance for a few years yet…

Rich had made the move from Canada to Ecuador to be a person of confidence for the company, to keep an eye on what was transpiring each day with the production plant. He had been sensitive as a young Lad or one that had visions of events that might come to pass. He, like many others with a gift, were afraid to continue receiving this information as the outcomes of some of these visions were real. For whatever reason Rich started to sleep on his stomach to stop these dreams or visions. As the dream body leaves through the umbilical or naval, then Rich's position for sleeping probably worked to cut the visions.

Traveler and Rishi did a Puja ceremony for Rich which helped to reopen his connection that he had suppressed in fear. During energy sessions or Reiki, he had some profound experiences that he could use as a base to continue on in his spiritual evolution if he chose that to be. In reality the energy work, Reiki or Pujas are a way to open up and receive guidance from your higher Self and from your guides, they have the wisdom to direct the energy to where it is needed.

During the Fall of 2010 Traveler and Rishi were coming to a point where they knew that this life of running a business would not be for a long period of time as it was taking them away from the life that they wanted to experience, one with more balance. In reality this work within the company was a great period of learning for them both, stretching them in many ways that cannot be done by living in the mountains or caves. It seems that the extremes in one's life are a necessity, experience them and then the pendulum returns to center. Extremes can be a benefit and if they are experienced, they are no longer a necessity in one's life. If a desire is suppressed then what you desire will most likely become stronger as your life continues to unfold, whether it's for exotic food, drink, sex, travel, more money or more material things etc., live them to the fullest and then return to a more balanced state of being, if that feels right to you. One makes a change in life when they are ready, the journey is theirs to discover.

Travel and Rishi decided to stay involved in the mining company for one more year. Traveler talked it over with Al to let him know that come September 2011 he would no longer work as manager/gerente of the company and Rishi would not be there to assist either. If Al was going to fill the position, he would need a translator and a person of confidence. They both agreed and felt that within a year there would be enough solid people in place to take care of the daily operation. One year seems like more than sufficient time when you are looking forward, but those months can pass quite quickly. Traveler and Rishi would be true to their word and most importantly loyal to their Self or Source…

One fine sunny morning Traveler suggested to Rishi and Victor that they should go to the beach called Baja Alto to meditate for a while and enjoy a day on the beach. Rishi is always ready for a new adventure, so they packed up the Land Cruiser and headed for the coast. Rishi had no idea what this day would bring. They arrived at the beach and walked until they found a quiet place away from the common beach area so they could light a few candles and incense to give gratitude to Mother Earth and their life experience. Within a few minutes the three of them sat quietly connecting, feeling the ocean breeze taking their thoughts away. Traveler did have one reoccurring thought that day, so he was probably the first one to come out of quiet time. When the moment was right Traveler went over to Rishi and kneeled before her in the sand and asked if she would like to be his wife or partner from this moment forward. Traveler did not have a ring but gave her a crystal as a symbol for this moment. Rishi was in tears and said, "En serio?"

Traveler took that as a yes. Victor enjoyed the moment as well. It was a special day indeed, not only to commit to each other but to their individual path home to Creator.

JUNGLE LIFE

If there is one thing constant in our experience here on Earth it is change and without it, one's life would shrivel up into complacency. The year 2011 would be the beginning of another level of change as well as a deeper search for answers. Rory, Nicole, and their daughter Lila made the move to Ecuador in January, here to stay for the next couple of years. Charlotte, Autumn, and Indra also arrived in Ecuador in February to experience life in this small but diverse country and to attend Traveler and Rishi's ceremony. This celebration would be a declaration to commit to a life of sharing their spiritual growth as a base to their life experience. All events would be looked at in relationship to spirit.

Their mining company had now attained a number of assets and work continued in preparation for the arrival of the processing plant from Africa and its installation. It was at this point where Al and Traveler had a chance to sell a few more shares of the company to those interested in a position with more involvement and direct ownership. It was with this blessing that Traveler and Rishi were able to purchase a 50-

hectare farm in the Oriente or Jungle area of Ecuador. This would become their home for the following two years.

This move to a remote property was in part being conscious of the date December 2012 which had caused much stir in the spiritual world. Nobody really knew what would happen and there were many people who just wrote the date off as another year like 2000 where everyone expected the computers of the world to shut down. Perhaps the world's economic platform or those individuals who have more influence on how information is exposed to the masses might have used this opportunity to cause a little more fear, and always the questions remain about the news, is it real or is it not... There are Hopis, Mayans and other Native people who are fairly accurate and/or in tune with the earth's changes, perhaps there is a miscalculation in the calendar, but the apex of the cycle has arrived. Our planet is not alone in this time of ascension or graduation to a new level of consciousness for humanity, this evolution is happening throughout our Universe.

This farm/jungle was definitely a gift from Source not only for the beauty of the area but for the raw connection to Mother Earth. The land sits on a plateau at about 1,000 meters above sea level and at the gateway to the great Amazon which extends out to the Atlantic Ocean through Brazil. There are four snow-capped volcanoes that are to the West and South of the farm, they are Sanguay, Altar, Chimborazo and Tungarauga. On a clear day with the blue skies in the background, there is a spectacular view of these majestic beings. Sanguay was the closest and is nothing short of awesome when it has a fresh blanket of snow on its peak.

This area is home to the Shuar Indians, who still retain ownership of much of this land. It would take a small book to describe the nature that is abundant in this paradise. There are Toucans painted with every color of the rainbow, flying about daily on the lookout for the next feed of seeds and fruits that the trees and plants have to offer. Everyday the skies are dotted with Eagles and Falcons soaring over the towering Pambil or Chonta, which are a palm tree that grows upwards of 30 meters high. Sometimes these majestic birds would swoop down near the houses to check out their new neighbors or perhaps rest in a nearby tree. There are black panthers, monkeys, and wild pigs to name a few and for those who like snakes, this is a haven for every color and every size. Streams flowing up out of the lush jungle floor, fast flowing rivers such as the Pastaza and eventually all flow joining the mighty Amazon. Pastaza river is a delight for any white-water enthusiast and extremely dangerous after a couple of days of rain. Any description of this area will fall short, only by living there for a while can one begin to capture an idea of what it has to offer…

It now was time to build a few houses and renovate the existing bungalow that was on the property. Traveler and Rishi selected a knoll sitting in the virgin Jungle alongside one of the streams and amongst the gigantic trees and flora. Rory and Nicole picked a hill more in the open with great views of the mountains and the driveway leading into the farm. Victor was on the highest point with Sanguay peering over his cabin. It was the existing bungalow that would serve as accommodations while the other houses were being built and later that year Charlotte and her family would come to live on the farm. It was a busy time as Traveler and Rishi were attending company affairs on the coast during the week and back to the farm on the weekends. It was wonderful to be back to the quiet solitude and take some time to give the workers a little guidance. They all had their nick names, Bamboo was the Jefe or foreman, Tigre was the youngest of the crew and Kata. Edgar was one of the three or four local Shuars, his name means dink in their language, he and his wife were hesitant to give the meaning, but they laughed afterwards. Jaime was nicknamed Hormiga which means ant because he never stops, and Victor was given the name Sambo who worked with them and quickly became good friends with the crew.

Building a house in the Jungle is not easy, most of the material was brought up by hand or by horse. After a few weeks, an extension to the driveway was built further into the farm which made the movement of material much easier. There was a small fire burning each day as the Shuar people use this method to keep the bats and insects out of their homes during and after construction. This method works for a while, but the old tradition had fires burning everyday inside the home for cooking, so the effect to ward off the bats continued to work.

The houses had a concrete base with hardwood floors laid over beams, Chonta was used for the upright columns as they become as strong as steel when cured. Studs were milled in Palora, and the exterior walls were made of bamboo taken from a grove on the farm. There is no doubt that the roof was one of the most interesting days of this construction. It is made of paja, a type of grass that grows in that area and probably throughout the Amazon, Edgar and his fellow Shuar were the experts and wrapped the paja on strapping almost like they were knitting. Upon completion this modern jungle home would look like many others in the neighboring Indigenous Villages with the only difference being that this one had electricity, hot and cold water with a pump and pressure system, bathrooms etc.… Life in the jungle was not all that difficult, ha ha.

Rishi and Traveler knew that the farm was for preparation which eventually they would come to understand what that word really meant in their lives, but not until a little later on. For now, they assumed that they were in preparation mode for the ongoing changes on earth and what those events would bring to the world. In any case they thought that they would be living on this property for a long time. Before long, a couple of cows were bought and soon the birth of two calves expanded the herd. There were a few goats and seven horses, actually starting to shape up as a farm. What would be a farm without a dog, seems like those numbers grew by the month. It was a wonderful environment for everybody and what a place for young children to grow up in, pure adventure…

Rory, Nicole, and Lila were still living on the coast close to the mining area as Rory was now preparing for the plant to arrive from Africa. This required the construction of a building, installation of the equipment and finally into production. By June of that year, Rishi had reached a point of not wanting to continue making the long haul back and forth to the coast each week, so she remained on the farm. It was a good decision as now she could keep a closer eye on construction. Traveler continued to make the nine-hour trip each week, he knew that it would eventually come to end.

Their farm had many lessons waiting for the family, some of them a little tough. Traveler's first one was the fact that Mother Nature was in her element in the Amazon and relentless in ability for continued growth. Back in Canada he was used to getting things in tip top shape, grass cut, trees trimmed and landscaping the yard to perfection. There was no chance in this lush jungle, with 4 meters of rain each year, the growth was uncontrollable. Traveler felt the anxiety and frustration of being helpless in his efforts to manage this awesome power of nature, it was the beginning of letting go of many things that caused tension in his life. It took a losing battle with nature in order for Traveler to realize that in order to be at peace he would have to recognize what the cause of tension was in his life. Let go and let life around you just be, find enjoyment in what life presents you, but do not become a slave to it.

Traveler had made his instructions clear, nice try but he was still short on conversing in Spanish. There were no shortages of trees in the jungle, but the boys were not to cut any of them unless they were instructed to do so. You have to laugh, they all smiled and nodded that they understood but apparently not. They needed beams and planks for construction of a small bridge and were used to cutting them out of the bush, why not, so close at hand. They asked Rishi if they could cut one tree, who in turn asked permission from Mother Earth and within a short period of time, the tree was selected. It was deep in the jungle, and you would never miss it.

Traveler returned home late that Friday afternoon and Rishi was a bit apprehensive but anxious to show him all the work that had been completed on their new home and of course the tour included the fallen tree. Traveler thought that nothing could rock the moment of happiness to be home and see Rishi again, but he still had some letting go to work on. When they reached the area where the tree lay on the jungle floor it was like Traveler had been numbed by some unknown force, he tried to rise above this energy and enjoy the moment with Rishi, but this energy was overwhelming. It took until the next day to finally accept the fact about the tree, rationalize the decision and let go. Rishi was clear in her mind, she had permission.

Traveler needed to begin to put life into perspective, sure there is too many stands of trees being cut in order to cultivate more farmland, but there was a time when harmony and balance was more prevalent between mankind and nature. Traveler loved hardwood floors just cut them somewhere else, not here. Eventually things rolled around into a better understanding and within a couple of days he was more willing to accept that he needed to give up some controlling issues in his life. He was still hard on the boys sometimes, especially Bamboo, misunderstanding and language barrier does not help. Bamboo had his experience, expertise and ideas, Traveler had his. In the end it is better to try and find some common ground, better to let go…

Rishi was getting more and more connected to Mother Earth, less in tune with time, and on the other side Traveler was still knee deep in a schedule, maybe a little higher than the knees. By September they were moved into their new home and construction was well under way on Rory and Nicole's home. It was time for Al's arrival and a trip to Cuenca to sign over the company. Al was now majority shareholder and Traveler resigned as gerente/manager and from here on out he would act as a consultant whenever needed. The rest of the Fall still required a bit of travel for meetings until Al was up to speed on the daily operation. Rory was still active in the company and remained until November when the Plant began producing its first concentrate.

One year had passed by and Al had now taken over the company. Traveler and Rishi would accept the outcome of their decision. They were looking for peace, yearning to know who they really are and begin to live life more in relationship to spirit, to be present as much as possible.

By this time Nicole and Lila were living on the farm and Rory was now making the commute whenever possible. It was time to begin exploring the Amazon region of Ecuador. Traveler and Rishi were interested in finding out how the Shuar were living and if they had maintained any sense of their ancestral ways. It was a time to return to the experience of more picnics by the river or near a waterfall. This little country has so much to offer and enjoy.

These long trips away from the farm for business became less and less desirable but they were still necessary. Palora is a small Village which is about 10 minutes from the farm gate. It was established in the early 1960s years and flourished with the founding of the Sangay Tea Estate in 1964. Sanguay Tea Estate has over five hundred hectares under management and still uses wood fires to dry the leaves.

One day Rory, Nicole, and Lila along with Traveler and Rishi were up on a hill where their meditation hut had been built. It was deeper into the farm and at the edge of the Jungle. This farm had twenty hectares of virgin Jungle and thirty hectares of pasture. They were all sitting on rocks and log seats near the Hut connecting to Mother Earth, just being quiet, when in a moment a flock of more than fifty large parrots and other birds flew directly over their heads and into the jungle. Before that moment passed a huge white Eagle flew in from the same direction, almost like it was herding the parrots towards the family. When the Eagle was in front of them it began to circle around and around up into the blue sky until it disappeared from site. They all just looked at one another and said, "Yep that was pretty special." Those are the moments that help bridge the gap between here and the unknown…

Rishi and Traveler's experiences in the Shuar communities were not what they were expecting. Having heard about the Yasuni tribe and their way of life they were expecting something similar, but not to be. Palora's Shuar community like many when civilization moves closer, became more interested in the outside world, life outside of their villages. They had become accustomed to alcohol, and many had a hard time adapting as they wanted to live like the folks in Palora but that meant that they had to leave most of their traditions behind. Traveler and Rishi came to know quite a few families from the Shuar community over the next couple of years and discovered that their life was not a whole lot different than any of the other locals. They were buying rice and other supplies in Palora and supplementing their diet with bananas, plantain and whatever else they could grow on their land. They had left their traditional ways many hundreds of years before. Traveler and Rishi were interested in ceremony, in living in complete harmony with nature, but maybe it was just a dream of days gone by.

Charlotte, Autumn, and Indra arrived in October and soon were adapting to life on the farm. Autumn and Indra continued with their habit of walking around barefoot, no thoughts about bugs. Most people who travel to Ecuador get their overdose of vaccines from the Doctor as a precaution to different bacteria here. These children were never vaccinated and are extremely healthy. In Traveler's time in school, they just lined all the students up in the hallway and gave everyone their shots, parents and students were oblivious to the harm these vaccines might cause.

There were lessons on the farm now available to experience. As a family of adults, they all had their individual lives, how would they blend that with three families living together. There was 50 hectares, lots of room, but everyone needed their privacy. They soon found out how far they were from unity consciousness, but they were all determined to resolve any issues. One base for the group became truth and transparency, don't be afraid to speak it, but you better be ready to live it. No more manipulation, it took a while to see how that was engrained into their lives. Truth brought about a couple of heated discussions but in the end they all learned from that moment and began to realize what it really takes to live in harmony. Their minds were the first target on the list, to try and get away from its habits as well as the emotions and memories that kept creeping up.

Traveler and Rishi had a little experience in this which began in Casacay, at least the first step of getting by that moment of a discussion where one just wants to walk away.

The questions between couples are many times the same ones, they never get answered because few are willing to stand there until the real cause or underlying problem arises. These problems are seldom caused by one or the other, it was some painful incident that got buried deep and with each painful moment during their life it either placed another layer of protection or accumulated another painful moment. These deep-seated memories are coming up to be liberated, accept that and be willing to go deep into your past and open up the way for these energetic patterns to be released. It takes guts and hard work, much easier to go outside and work in the garden. Be truthful and transparent, and from there pain can be replaced by a feeling of freedom and lightness of heart once again. Truth can be hurtful sometimes, but it is the true liberator.

During their time on the farm Rishi and Traveler used to bike into Palora and some days they would head in the other direction to a small village called the Diez y Seis de Agosto, close to the neighboring Shuar community. It was early on in their relationship when Traveler first met Rishi that he had asked Creator, if it were possible, that he would take some of Rishi's karma or pain. He can honestly say, "be careful what you ask for." She had had a more than difficult life from Traveler's point of view and wanted to help in some way. A few times it happened that Traveler felt similar pain along with Rishi but normally not too severe. On this day they were riding their bikes into Diez y Seis, enjoying the breeze as they felt like they were flying going down the hill. They had picked up quite a bit of speed and Rishi had both hands up in the air like wings, Traveler thought maybe that was not a good idea, but he had his own moment to ride. Rishi was nearing the bottom of the hill, hands on the bars once again, when the front wheel spun to the left and she went flying off, landing on the bike and finally the pavement. Traveler was calm but was concerned that she had hurt herself. Rishi got up off the road laughing, not a mark on her body, they were good to go. They had stopped to visit a family in the village, and it was about twenty minutes later when Traveler felt like he had been hit by a truck, it was a numbness that vibrated from his bones. It lasted for a few hours, long after they were back home. Maybe it was a coincidence but not likely.

As part of their ongoing search of the truth they spent some time with a Shaman and his son who had been initiated into Shamanism. Juan was living his period of purification which was one year of not eating meat and no sexual relationships. He was committed to staying focused on his father's teachings which had been passed down from their ancestors. It was with the permission of the elder Shaman (grandfather) that they decided to open up their sacred ceremonial caves to those people interested in experiencing an Ayahuaska Ceremony. There are many petrified forms on this property, a large snake head, turtle and other forms leading into the cave. Rishi and Traveler set a night aside for their ceremony in this sacred cave, anxious to see what their experience would be.

It was late at night as they followed the Shaman and his wife down along the rock pathway lit up by the moon. When they reached the entrance to the cave they needed to descend between the boulders and then off to the left was the mouth of this sacred space.

Their guiding moon had long since slipped behind the boulders, leaving them in absolute darkness. As they found their way to the ceremonial site, a candle was lit so they could begin to set up their herbs and flowers. Everyone found their place to sit and prepare. You could feel the energy of the past resonating from the walls, a tradition of ceremony somewhere between mystical and myth. This elder Shaman cleansed their energies with herbs and then he began to share the Ayahuaska blend. Rishi and Traveler managed to drink a small glass and the Shaman drank a fair bit more, trying to reach a certain state. They all had some good visions entering their mind space and the Shaman was quite satisfied to get confirmation from Rishi on a few images or energies that they had witnessed.

Later that evening, once Rishi and Traveler were asleep the lucid dreams were upon them, just as the Shaman said might happen. Traveler found himself in an open pasture with a couple of trees and one huge black bull with exceptionally long horns. It was a dream, but this bull seemed real and snorting in anger. Luckily, the dream provided a rope with which Traveler quickly tied the bull's legs together and secured it to the tree. Now that the bull was safely out of the way, Traveler went to sleep for the rest of the night. They were staying in a small Hosteria in the Jungle, so the conditions were ideal for rest.

Early the next morning they returned to the Shaman's family home for tea and breakfast. He and Juan began to decipher the meanings of these dreams and put their perspective on them. As they were sharing their thoughts, they explained that this was the way that they began each day, talking about their dreams from the night before. It was from their dreams that they took guidance on how to experience the day ahead of them, paying attention to the signs given them.

There was one last part of the ritual or tradition to perform and that was a cleansing from the fresh water in a stream nearby. It was quite cool, but it did feel liberating once the purification was completed. Traveler and Rishi invited them to the farm to perform a ceremony with Charlotte and Nicole which they agreed to.

When the day finally came the Shaman arrived with his wife and son Juan. They spent most of the day walking along the jungle path, learning about the different medicinal plants growing on the farm. Much to their surprise there were many plants that could be eaten and others that could be used for energy cleansing. Their Ayahuaska experience was memorable but not a tradition that they wanted to pursue any further on their personal journeys.

Not long into 2012 Traveler and Rishi loaded up their backpacks and headed for Puerto Morona on the Peruvian border entering into the Amazon. They were still searching for a traditional tribe that lived each day connected to Mother Earth and Father Sun. They spent a couple of days in this village watching the boat traffic that was transporting people and goods, some guided by Indigenous, and some were commercial vessels, taking supplies into remote areas. This network of Rivers is still the Pastaza that runs not so far from their farm. They finally contacted an Ecuadorian man named Victor. He rarely wore a shirt and seemed right at home in the Jungle and most importantly was known for his guiding abilities throughout this area.

Victor is a small statured man with a sparse beard, kind of looked like a younger Miyagi, long ponytail and particularly good natured. Traveler and Rishi made arrangement to rendezvous the following morning and walk into his property which was located along the river.

Early the next morning Victor and his son lead them along a path to the river, Traveler and Rishi were quick to catch on that they needed to pack lighter next time, as their backpacks were close to forty lbs. They set up their tents, dug a hole for the bathroom facility, lit a fire and were ready for lunch, all in the space of about two hours. Victor was accustomed to cooking and took his guiding work seriously, so it was a very relaxing few days. That afternoon Victor spoke with a couple of the Shuar neighbors who had canoes with motors and selected the bigger canoe to take them to a remote Shuar village the next day. This village was in Peru and the trip would require them to stop at a couple of Military check points who monitored movement back and forth from the two countries. They also would need permission from the Tribe to enter their village and with hope that they could spend the night. This is something that is discussed by the Tribe's elders and not always guaranteed entry.

Traveler washed up in the river that afternoon, as did Victor and his son, pretty sure there were piranhas, but he kept close to shore just in case there was a siting.

Their group headed out next morning, ready for adventure, quiet a trip on this immense river that winds its way to the East through Brazil. This river is home to pods of pink dolphins known as Botos, unfortunately they are a target practice for some of the military. If time were taken out of the equation this trip could have been taken hundreds of years before and looked exactly the same. Not much had changed for many families living along the riverbank, with their homes of dirt floors, bamboo walls and a paja roof. Part of this area was a battlefield when Peru and Ecuador were at war over border territory. The Ecuadorian president at that time gave up a lot of Ecuadorian land to Peru in order to stop the slaughter of men, so it is written. He promptly left the country with a fair stash of cash; many Presidents from Ecuador have had a similar exit, to start a new life in another country.

After a full day traveling this scenic river, they arrived at the banks of their destination and pulled up to the docks. Victor and the Shuar owner of the canoe were greeted by one of the Elders (Anciano) who took them up to the village where they would sit together and discuss whether permission to stay would be given. Victor had spent a year living with the Yasuni Tribe in Ecuador, so he knew what etiquette was required. Traveler and Rishi stayed on the banks of the river trying to make friends with the children, but the little ones were cautious. Victor returned smiling, with a couple of villagers alongside him to welcome our group to their village, all was good…

This remote village was rather impressive as they had built a walkway coming up from the river and it continued around a couple of spring fed ponds where a few families were washing their clothes. They continued up the trail until they reached the village up on the hill. It was well laid out with sufficient space between each home which were built from wood, bamboo and paja. There was never a shortage of building material in the Jungle. In an open space they had paja hanging on a line to be dried, preparing it for use on a new roof or for reparations. There were a few bathrooms in amongst the bushes here and there, basically a hole in the ground with a bit of concrete around it and bamboo walls for a bit of privacy. It was decided that Traveler and Rishi would stay with one family where they would provide meals for them.

Once the introductions were made and they were settled in, they walked around the village to meet a few other families. This village was well laid out giving each family their own sense of property. It was not too long into the walk when they encountered the source of laughter which was one neighbor's home which was a gathering place, apparently this family had the secret recipe for good tasting Chicha (fermented yuca or corn). This group was well into storytelling and laughing, no work today. Many traditional tribes made their Chicha with chewed Yuca, the women of the tribe would chew the Yuca and then spit it into the drum or pail and then let this liquid ferment. This particular Chicha appeared to have some kick to it as they were well under the effects. After a while it was time for Rishi and Traveler to return to their guest family so that they could share a few stories over supper. It was a simple meal, a chicken leg soup with yuca and another yuca on a side plate. It would suffice for the night, and it was well appreciated.

Somewhere during their walk, it was decided by the Chief that Rishi and Traveler would spend the night in his home and learn more about their ways with his family. Not your usual remote area tribal home. It had a running generator so that they could all watch TV or play music, not the beat of the drum, more like rap. Traveler and Rishi sat and talked with the Chief for a couple of hours during which time he talked about his role as a high school professor in a small city in Peru. It is his experience in the outside world that gave him the ideas to share with his family and village. He was at that time lobbying the government to bring in electricity to his village, there was no road, just travel on the river. His family, more than the others in the village were dressed in more fashionable clothing, quite a different feeling in their presence.

It was soon time for bed, Traveler and Rishi were given a space on the floor in the kitchen, not so bad for one night, only Traveler was a little weary that the cats might have missed a rat or two on their watch. The Chief had his own out-house in the backyard, so it was not too far to find your way if it became necessary to make the trip during the night.

The next morning it was up early, no problem letting your feet hit the floor… After breakfast they would be back on the river heading home to Victor's property. Breakfast was served in the same family home where they had eaten supper and this meal consisted of yuca and a boiled egg. Keeping a trim figure would not be a problem. It was time to say thank you, gather their bags and head out. Traveler and Rishi left a bit of money to help the family who had shared their home and hospitality as they said their good-byes.

There really was not much to learn from the village as they were being influenced by the Chief, who had modernization and a better life in mind. It is a tough call as to whether modernization really would benefit the tribe, but as the famous Sage Ramana Maharshi often said, "It is as it is." Traveler and Rishi were more intent in learning more about ceremony and the Tribe's connection to Mother Earth, but it appeared that those traditions were slowly disappearing generation by generation.

Many from the village walked down to the Dock to say goodbye, the children were now more willing to express their playful side and performed along the banks of the river. Rishi and Traveler waved good-bye and the canoe motored out and away on their trip upriver. On their trip the day before they had a chance to cruise up one of the river's tributaries where they had watched a hundred or so piranhas feeding on top of the water. They can definitely move at the speed of light. The trip back would not be conducive to meandering as the torrential rain began about mid-way point. After a half hour or so of this downpour they finally gave up on the idea of staying dry. This rain seemed to be ideal for the pink dolphins, so they made an appearance on one of the bends along the river, so it was well worth getting wet.

Once Traveler and Rishi were back on shore at Victor's they changed into some dry clothes and got ready to watch Victor and his son, harvest Makundi. This larva starts out as an insect egg laid in a rotting Chonta or other species of tree trunk. They gathered up about 50 of these thumb sized grubs and figured that would be more than enough to sample. Victor got a fire going and prepared the Makundi for the frying pan so that everyone could try this jungle delicacy. These little snacks were quite tasty, and it was wonderful to see what earthly treasures one could enjoy.

Once again, the next morning Traveler and Rishi packed up their gear and headed back to Puerto Morona where they would spend another night. The scenery from this small river port back to Palora is quite breathtaking but Sanguay always stands out as absolutely spectacular. The road near the city of Macas passes quite close to Sanguay and the Volcano keeps one's attention for a long while, sitting like an ancient white capped mystic connection to the past.

Once they were back on the farm a decision was made to spend more time focused on their center, heart area or seat of their soul. Rishi was living from her heart more and more each day, Traveler was still skating around more with the mind and having a rather difficult time trying to discover his center, not like it was so far away. They had been practicing celibacy since December 2011, willing to do whatever it took to focus all energy inward towards Self.

Traveler and Rishi started to spend many days at a time in silence and some of those days were also set aside for no physical touch or eye contact. The latter can really get the mind smoking as it is always looking for security and confirmation that their relationship was going well, but eventually the mind quiets and trust becomes absolute. Their clock was disconnected, trying to eliminate the habit of living in tune with time and schedules. Does time exist? Well for this experience on Earth it appears so, probably a necessity to have a chance to rejuvenate these physical bodies.

They changed their eating habits as well, down to two meals a day, this was an easy adapt for Rishi as she had been through fasts many times in her life, some by choice, some not. Traveler still had his morning coffee to keep hunger at bay until 9:30 or so, and that had been quite an accomplishment to break the habit of eating breakfast around 7:00 o'clock every morning, that might have been engrained during his early days on the family farm.

It was a time of trying to break habits, change **beliefs** and begin to clear memories that were affecting their daily lives and interfering with their connection to Source. Can this healing be done without breaking the habitual way of life? Perhaps, but you really have to shake the mind out of its nest or perch, in order to regain control of your experience of life and truly make conscious decisions on how you want to live it.

During their first few days of silence Traveler decided to try and put the mind and body to rest by sitting on the couch and just watching the thoughts without acting on any. It was like sitting on a wild tomcat, within a few minutes the mind wanted to go outside and pick a few leaves for tea, or make a tea, or go to the bathroom, or clean the kitchen it never really quit but it was during this time that Traveler began to see the mind's patterns. Ever so slowly becoming more aware of the mind's potential and begin to take back control of his own experience.

Our minds have no concept of future nor any capacity to view it, at least not directly but it spends a lot of time out there planning and away from enjoying the present moment. It can only retrieve information out of the past memories, no wonder humans repeat and repeat life situations, no way out if the mind is at the wheel and driving your experience.

Journey Home

This mystery that seems to elude much of humanity is yet so close at hand. How could any attempt made by the mind to accumulate knowledge have any significance in comparison to all that you already are? Imagine those times when you are sitting alone in nature, the mind is quiet, and you are present to that moment. There is no search required in those blissful moments, it is your true nature. A walk in nature for sure is a wonderful home base but it is necessary to remove the harmful patterns and beliefs that are blocking out our connection to Source. How wonderful is the idea to be Life rather than all that work of trying to live it?

Imagine a moment in the depths of a big city where horns are honking, power lines buzzing, people chatting or screaming, dogs barking and sirens wailing. It is definitely more of a challenge for one's spiritual advancement if the mind is fully engaged to the outside world. It is more than enough that the mind is using all the old habits, beliefs, relationships, memories etc. to project itself into the future and set up the next experience. Many times, a person moves to a new part of the country or to another country to try and get away from the circumstances that seem to be negatively affecting their life experience, only to find out that the circumstances return, Traveler had a first-hand glimpse of that.

It has been repeated by many a Guru over the past thousands of years that the place to start on the journey home to Source is to quiet the mind. Yes, for many it is not an easy task, but that does not mean that you should give up on the idea. Humanity often seems to take the easier path, sometimes painful but at least they know what to expect. It is similar to the story of the hound dog laying on the front porch enjoying the Summer breeze. Only one irritant in this dog's life at the moment was the nail that he was lying on. This hound dog would lift his body up a bit every once in a while, and bay in discomfort to anyone that would listen but then quickly return to rest on that nail, it was just not worth the effort to get up and move away from the pain.

One has to make themselves available for Creator to come into their life or make time to connect to that fragment of Divine Light that is in union with your soul, never letting you out of site. If you stay the course, you will eventually integrate with this fragment or Thought Adjuster that accompanies all souls on their adventures.

Once again it is not easy as we are distracted with our daily experience or the activities outside and remain connected there. Meditation is certainly a key and if scheduled into each day, the practice can help bring your experience into balance and so much more. Remember, your connection is always there, never leaving you for a second, but it is up to each individual to consciously be in connection and then be a witness to the peace that comes into your life experience. Your choice, your decision.

Traveler was blessed to have time in his life to make this concentrated effort and wake up from his daily norm. It was after a couple of days being focused on the task at hand which meant being quiet on the couch, that something changed. Traveler was sitting there early one evening listening to flute music by Manose Singh and within a short time his upper body started to move in a rhythmical dance. His arms were making exact movements up and down the chakras, in and around the front of the body. It felt like an active meditation, so he just let go to the moment. Rishi and Victor were out on the porch, observing once and a while with a little smile but Traveler was oblivious to all else…

One never knows what the next day will bring but this one was the beginning of a deeper or more meaningful change in Traveler's experience. He was sitting in quiet time, before the sun came up, no speculation just being conscious. In a moment he felt his arms going into prayer position in front of his heart and from there his hands were connecting meridian points and spiraling up with energy. During this time, he was speaking another language, one that he didn't understand. Near the end of this session Traveler or this moment said, "I am Ushkikywa." It was repeated several times so he could remember it when quiet time was over. There was quite a feeling of gratitude for Great Spirit which was expressed in words at the end. Traveler was a little dumb founded but yet excited to the possibility that this perhaps was his soul's name. The morning was spent enjoying this lucid moment which lasted for a few hours and sharing it with Rishi.

It would be clear the following morning that this name was not Traveler's soul name but only one of the many experiences that he had had on Mother Earth. Over the next three and half months or so these meditations continued to reveal other life experiences with different languages such as different native Tribes, Gaelic, French, Asian and others not recognizable. There were two others that he feels are language of light and the other known as a language of the gods.

Each day was over an hour and a half in morning meditation or in trance like Ceremony, it was becoming evident that many previous lifetimes had been of a spiritual nature as there was much knowledge on the energy channels of the physical body and energetic bodies. In almost every afternoon during this time period other Ceremony type meditations took place. There were facial designs that were learned some mornings, and these were painted on Traveler's face by Rishi using moistened ashes. Many times, there was a specific smudging done in the house before ceremonies began, using palo santo, garlic leaves, sage, rosemary etc. There were a number of ceremonies done in honor of Mother Earth or Mahii, all given in a great feeling of gratitude.

There was one afternoon that was different from all others, it was a re-enactment of somewhere around twenty-five deaths from different lifetime experiences. There were quite a number of deaths done by dragging the body with a horse. That was creative... One of the deaths was of what seemed to be a witch or someone knowledgeable in the occult, no fear was felt in the body during any of the deaths that surfaced.

Traveler felt the need to stop these experiences, one reason was they were putting quite a drain on his body's energy and second, he wanted to make sure that the mind/ego had not jumped in at some point to claim the experiences. It was early on during these three and a half months that Traveler had had a vision. He saw himself standing by a small leafy tree near the corner of their home with a shovel in his hand. He shared the vision with Rishi, and she suggested that he go to the spot and sit quietly to get a sense of where to dig. Rishi was close by sitting on Mia, a being who has inhabited a big rock close to their home for over a million years. This place from the vision was located and with Mother Earth's permission Traveler began to dig a hole near the small tree.

He and Rishi carefully removed each stone and before long they came to realize that it was a small burial site. There were pebbles, small stones, and pieces of ceramic, simple things that they tried to keep in order as they were removed. It was during the time that Traveler was digging that Rishi had an Indian woman dressed in white come into her 3rd eye vision. She began to communicate through her heart, asking Rishi, "What is he doing?" referring to Traveler. Rishi replied that Traveler was following a vision that he had had. The Indian woman said, tell him to stop digging when he finds what he is looking for.

Rishi gathered up the pebbles and ceramic pieces in a pot and Traveler stopped after he encountered a red colored stone which was a bit larger than a golf ball. It was a rust-colored red with quite a few soft spots that were cream colored. Off they went to wash the little treasures inside the house.

It was during that moment that Rishi started to receive information from Ninfa. She spoke about a time 800 years before when a holy child had been born among their Tribe, Ninfa was his mother. Traveler, during that lifetime was the spiritual leader for their Tribe. This young child even at two years of age had a high level of conscious and was the long-awaited gift to help bring their Tribe into a higher understanding or consciousness. It was beyond comprehension at that time, but this young boy made a conscious decision to leave this plane and allow the death of his young mortal body.

It was tradition for their Tribe to have the mother of this holy child, accept death in gratitude for this gift that was bestowed upon them. Their holy child would grow up teaching them the ways or understanding of a greater connection to Source and how to govern their community. After this child's death, his mother and Tribe were devastated, not only for her son's death but their loss of direct spiritual guidance. It became known to Rishi and Traveler, that it was Traveler who had laid the child to rest in this small grave as part of a ceremony with the Tribe over eight hundred years prior.

These stones, pebbles and pieces of ceramic were the original offerings, many of which were now sitting on the kitchen counter in their home. There was a group of sacred stones in amongst this collection. Ninfa gave instructions on which stones they were and out of that selection Traveler was asked to select the four primary stones representing North, South, East, and West. These stones, if used properly could answer questions of a spiritual nature. Ninfa said that Traveler had to initiate Rishi on these stones as he was the original teacher that taught her so long ago. Traveler went into a trance like state and preformed a ceremony with Rishi to initiate her on the use of the sacred stones. The stones were used over the next couple of years now and then were given a new home in Lake Titicaca in Peru. There are some things in life that just cannot be explained.

In order to complete their work, the next morning Traveler and Rishi performed a ceremony to place the remaining articles back into the burial site. Nearing the end of the ceremony Traveler and Rishi could see over a hundred Natives dressed in white standing in celebration at the bottom of the hill and as well Ninfa closer to the burial site. It was a very emotional moment for Traveler as memories were released and healing was completed for him as well as for the Tribe.

Creation is for the most part beyond the concept of our three-dimensional mind and it is difficult to have an understanding of life playing out simultaneously, past, present and future. As Mother Earth continues on her ascension path, our planet requires healing, as does the human race and all life forms here. Self- healing requires work, and since humanity has free will it is up to each one to do their own healing which includes cleaning out the memories and beliefs affecting our physical and emotional health. This process is so important to all of humanity, without this effort how will we ever live-in harmony with each other.

It is through this healing process that a soul truly begins to live in peace, in harmony with it's brothers and sisters throughout creation. For those who are unsure where to begin there are many qualified Healers on Mother Earth at this time who can assist in this process or be a guide to liberate these memories. Once the interference that these habits and memories cause, begin to be cleared then our true nature or peaceful state begins to shine through, and our perspective on life changes, more loving, more Human.

In the beginning of November that year, Charlotte, Autumn, and Indra were on a plane and heading home to Canada where they would continue on with their experience. Rory had moved to Quito along with Nicole and Lila, as he was now working with his cousin and Uncle Rod. A son was born to Rory and Nicole near the end of November, a new grandson for the Clan on both sides of the families. As their experience in the Amazon was coming to a close the farm was listed for sale with a realtor.

Rishi and Traveler had spent some time in Pifo with Rory and his family and then they moved to Manta on the coast until the end of the year. When they returned to the farm in the new year, they begin to wonder why the property had not sold yet. It did not take too long before they realized that the family had performed a ceremony in gratitude for Mother Earth and had asked the Arch Angels to protect their farm.

There was a circle of stones still located at the end of the driveway near their house which had been placed for the original ceremony. Rishi had received information that another ceremony was needed to release the farm in order that a new family could take over. This ceremony that was required was a little more in detail as they would be opening the way for the new owners to actually make the purchase. Pedals of flowers were dropped on both sides of the driveway which was close to 500 meters long as well as the entrance to each house along the way. Another formation of stones was placed in the form of the Star of David with an entrance stone placed to the South as that was the direction of Traveler and Rishi's next move. The ceremony was completed as instructed and within five days they received a call from the Agent saying that an interested party would be arriving within a week. This family from the USA purchased the farm and soon Rishi & Traveler would be in search for their new home and next experience.

Part of the shift to a life experience with Spirit as your guide, is believing in that fact of Its existence, and the more you have faith or trust in that connection and power within you, the grander your experience with Spirit is.

Samuel McLeod

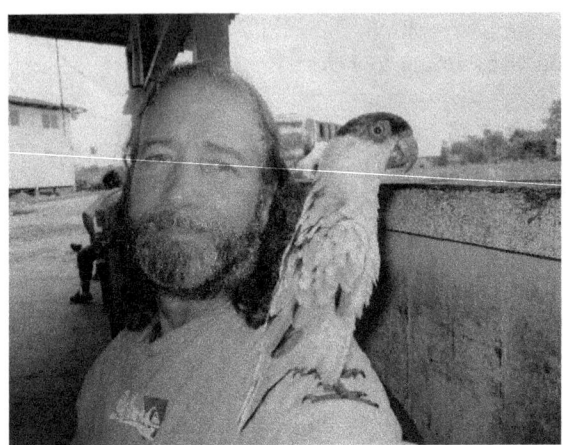

SOUTHERN CROSS

The property in Palora had come in a vision or dream to Rishi, the next place was to be found by being in their hearts; that was a little vague, but they had a name of Elvira as a point to begin. It is not even a Pueblo but did exist not too far from Vilcabamba which is Southern Ecuador. If there is a perfect climate to be experienced, it is in this part of Ecuador close to the border of Peru.

Rishi and Traveler spent a few days looking at properties throughout this area and then further North near Malacote, in the province of Loja. Any property that they put an offer on either was not accepted or by the time the seller had decided to accept, Rishi and Traveler had decided against the purchase. One day as they were waiting for their Vehicle to be cleaned up, they were reading the classified ads and found a farm for sale near Peru which was further West towards the coast. They called the owner and by mid-day they were walking the farm. It has a beautiful valley to the West with a ridge of Andes backing and surrounding this picturesque view from the entrance of this property. Rishi and Traveler sat on the ground for a while and felt the peace seeping up through their bodies. They were pretty sure but wanted to give the decision one more night to let it sink in. The next morning, they were greeted by the deep blue skies above the farm with a gentle breeze giving perfect essence to the moment, no further coaxing required, they arrived at a price and the search was over.

Within a short time, they were settled into an apartment in the nearby village of Catacocha and waiting for the building crew from Palora to arrive. Bamboo had agreed to spend a few months with them and build another home for Traveler and Rishi. It was a long way from the Jungle area where he lived but he was anxious for a new project. He brought Tigre and Momo along with him. Victor was happy to be reunited with his friends and all were looking forward to getting started. Soon the backhoe was clearing a spot for the garage and house; this site was close to the dirt road so there was easy access for material to arrive. The climate from June to November is normally dry in this area, warm and with a nice breeze so it was a perfect time of year for construction.

It was a wonderful time building this house, no long trips each week, just a 10-minute drive up the mountain road to for supplies. The new home was built using brick for the walls with an open beam ceiling. The roof was laid with teja, an old-style ceramic. It is great for this area as the teja roof does not allow the sun to penetrate inside the house. Floors were laid with dark terra cotta tile, to offset the salmon brick color. Traveler and Rishi were trying to build with as many natural materials as possible, keeping a good connection with Mother Earth. Their bed frame was made with brick with the opening going straight down to the earth. This was filled with a spiral of placed stones and a number of crystals; their bed had a seat built into the brick and as well the mattress laid over the rocks.

Water was piped down from the mountain so there would be no need for electricity or pumps. A wind generator was to be

Journey Home

installed but the supplier faulted on his import paperwork, so the unit was held up at Customs in Guayaquil.

Living without electricity really was not too difficult to adapt to, there was gas cooking and good pressure on running water. Most nights the moon lights up the sky so one could still walk around outside and if the need arose there was still the gas generator which was used during construction. Rishi and Traveler had slept above the storage area in the garage for the last month of construction, they wanted to enjoy the experience of those moonlit nights as well as the nature that abounds in this area. They could see the Southern Cross so clearly as it set itself over the top of the mountain each night. It was wonderful to see light beings flash down across the mountain close to their house. There are few neighbors, and many do not have electricity, so the ambiance was perfect to witness these beings.

Our minds can be limiting but Creation has no limits, many beautiful things exist all around us, even in this time space. Some children are still open to see things, like a Fairy, but as parents are in disbelief soon the child accepts this new fact, that it is just imagination. Become like children and believe.

By late September it was time for Bamboo, Momo and Tigre to head back to the Oriente, it had been a great Summer for everyone. Traveler had decided to head up to Canada for a few months to work with Rory who had returned home seven months prior. Traveler and Rishi had run the budget a little tight and it appeared that going to Canada would help fill the coffers once again. Traveler and Rishi never like being apart, not even for a moment, it is a feeling that is difficult to describe but they miss each other sometimes even though they are at each other's side. They had a good cry the night before heading to the Airport and both were ready for the challenge ahead, that of being apart.

Canada is beautiful but the area in and around Vancouver is breath taking. Rory was waiting at the Airport for Traveler and within a few minutes they were having lunch and getting caught up once again. The rest of the afternoon was spent at the jobsite getting acquainted with everybody before starting the next morning. After a short afternoon it was an hour ride to the house. It was certainly wonderful to see Nicole, Lila, and Esca once again.

While Traveler was on the farm in Palora he had heard the voice once again one morning during quiet time, it said, "Have no fear, I am here to look after you, even to wash the body." It took a little while to catch onto, the wash the body part of the message but after a while Traveler had a fairly good notion that it meant purification.

Healing the body takes a sincere effort of clearing up memories, beliefs and habits and it does not happen over-night. Just when you think that anger or another emotion has been cleared up, you head into town only to find that the next person who cuts in front of you in the line-up, has somehow become your teacher and brought the evil one to the surface once again. If you can stay the course and remain focused each time an emotion such as anger arises, you become a little more aware of the whole event. It is not easy to take a few deep breaths and see that the problem is within you, something inside of you that is being trigged by another person. It requires a little more compassion for your brother/sister in front of you and for yourself. If you are open and awake these moments can truly be an opportunity to let go. Traveler had had a pretty peaceful Summer, energy on the farm was great, hardly a blip along the way.

Traveler is quite sure that Creator has a wonderful sense of humor, ah yes, I'll even wash your body, as each day something or someone is placed in your path to help with the proverbial bathing. It took a couple of weeks to get into the rhythm of work, Rory and Traveler were heading out the door with coffee in hand around 5:30 every morning and getting home around 6 o'clock in the afternoon.

During the first few weeks Traveler was looking after the temporary workers brought in to help with clean up on the site. Traveler had been living more like a Monk, nobody really bothering him until now… For the most part these workers were all fairly good, but the odd one could get a rise out of Traveler. Once again, he felt the heat rising within his jacket as David or Robert would have problems keeping order in the garbage bin, now that is a serious problem, yeh… right. Was control still a bit of an issue that needed clearing?

Traveler was soon smiling at his re-action to these workers, relax and let go. It was not long before Traveler realized that one of the real reasons he was in Canada, was in part for his ongoing mastery of his emotions, and to work at cleaning up habits and releasing memories. Each day now became a chance to be more aware, pay attention to the moment and what was passing by, more in observation. Definitely not everyone has a chance to do their spiritual work on the quiet of a farm, it is a blessing, and then have an opportunity to test out the work off the farm, to see if the peaceful feeling is real. Traveler had a way to go but awareness was settling in to stay.

It was a wonderful time to be able to share each day with Rory and compare spiritual notes at the end of the day or just laugh at the craziness of it all. Most days it was a cappuccino for the ride home and the odd time a brownie or date square, Traveler wasn't completely into purifying the body just yet, still time to enjoy the dulces (sweets) of this world. Living in Canada would probably be a little more difficult to become detached to all the conveniences, the great tasting food, clean streets, well organized Urban living, recreational parks, lakes, rivers etc. but on the other hand Ecuador is a perfect environment for getting rid of desires at least it was for Traveler.

Back home Rishi was deeper into her own process in many ways. Victor liked sleeping over at his friend's family home, so Rishi had lots of time to get over any fear of being alone. Being alone can also bring up a lot of things from within and there is nowhere to run, they have to be dealt with. She was connecting more and more with Mother Earth and with her higher Self or her true Self. She had worked hard on staying centered or living in her heart and now the flow of information and guidance from within was growing each day. Traveler and Rishi had much to share but the phone connections were rarely good, so they would have to wait until Traveler returned home in December and get caught up on the last three months. It was during these few months that Mother Earth placed three vortexes on the property, one was centered in the garage, one in the living-room of their home and one down by the Mango tree. These three vortexes formed a triangle and Rishi was able to witness the increase in strength of each one and the eventual connection of the three. Their purpose would be known later on.

Traveler's workplace continued to be an opportunity to clear memories as they arose. It is not always possible in this environment to be able to stop work for a moment or two, but Traveler did whenever time permitted. When a feeling arises such as self-doubt, shame, blame, guilt, or a feeling of not being good enough, it is in that moment that one needs to feel this energy and be with it, totally.

Close your eyes and ask to see the moment (memory) that caused this feeling which was recorded in your subconscious. When that moment comes up, it may be when you were a child or teenager, only you will know. For example, the memory comes up that an older brother said that you are just a baby, or get out of here and leave me alone, or your mother is having an off day and takes her frustration out on you with a cuff on the ear. Whatever the moment is you need to return to it and sit with yourself (the child, teenager, or adult that you were at the time), sit with that moment, give yourself love and also give love to those who were part of that moment. Let go of the misunderstanding of that moment, as you give it love, feel this energy dissolving and send it back to Mother Earth in the form of light flowing into a pond or river that might be close by. Ask Mahii/Gaia to bring this moment into harmony, balance, and peace. There may be other memories attached with this feeling, some that go deeper and some you will not think were related, accept them without judgment, give them love and let go. It takes time and patience, until the feeling has no power over you and eventually leaves you. Only you can do this work. Purification is returning to the child like state, open to experience the adventures of the moment, empty to receive the flow of life, no speculation.

Another way for clearing memories or unwanted habits in your life is to take time to sit by a fire. Build the fire and use it as a ceremony of gratitude, with flowers, fruits, rice etc. as an offering to Mahii, Tata Inti and Great Spirit or God. As you sit or stand by the fire, visualize the intention (of what you want to let go off) rising up as a ball of energy in your heart area or heart chakra, once the intention is set, move the energy down to your base chakra. Continue to build this ball of energy in your base chakra and when you feel that it is time, let the ball of energy (your intentions) flow up through your chakras and out your crown and into the fire to be dissolved and brought back into peace, harmony and balance. This can also be used to sever energetic ties with old relationships. Use the fire to clean out any items in your home that are no longer being used, these things can also hold unwanted energy. Whatever words you have for making a change in your life, speak them to the fire, ask for your guides to be more active in your life, give them permission to assist you. You are a sacred being, take these moments to claim your sovereignty and connect to your cosmic brothers/sisters and most importantly to that Fragment of Source (Thought Adjuster) that is eternally with you.

Autumn was passing by quickly and it would be soon time to return to Ecuador. The last day of work with Rory arrived; Traveler had become accustomed to the daily commute and also spending time with his fellow workers, but it had come to completion. Traveler wanted to spend the December Solstice with Rishi and as well the rare cross formation of Jupiter, Venus, Mars, and Mercury would be brilliant in the evening sky on the farm. Traveler made plans to visit Charlotte who was now living on Maui. He landed on the Island and remembered its beauty, it had been 33 years since he had vacationed there with his brother Hugh, G and Fran.

Charlotte came to the Airport with Autumn and Indra to greet her father. Traveler was excited to see them again, a lot of time had passed since they left the farm in Palora in 2011. There was a good long hug for everyone and then back to their home to get caught up. Traveler was hoping to meet with some of the Hawaiian people who had maintained their connection to Mother Earth and asked Charlotte if there existed any on Maui. She said that many or most were just busy with life and trying to make a living, more or less like much of humanity they had slowly forgotten the ways of their Elders or did not have time to practice it in their life experience. There are some traditional tribes on other Islands in Hawaii but there would not be an opportunity to meet them on this trip.

Autumn was attending a more traditional school and was learning the Hawaiian language. It was a treat to listen to all the students sing in their native language out on the lawn before beginning their classes. Indra took the opportunity to explore the playground while he was waiting for his mom.

One day they loaded up the SUV and drove around the coast. There was time for a barbeque on the beach and a splash in the ocean. They stopped later that day at a very mystical place where the coastline was filled with natural rock arches and designs jutting up from the Sea. The surf splashed high into the sunlight, freeing the mind, and letting it surrender to being present. In one of the nearby caves, Traveler caught the movement of some energy darting back and forth. He took 4 or 5 photos with his camera and on one shot he had captured the light body of a Fairy, quite in detail. Too busy making a living to make a life really seems true in moments like this. If we do not take the time to connect to Source, then we will miss a lot of what Life has to offer us in our experience here on Earth.

Traveler was soon saying good-bye once again and then on his way back to Vancouver to spend a day shopping before his return home. It was interesting to see how their small family was out experiencing life in their own way. Each one, discovering their self through the highs and lows, the happiness and sadness, the quiet and the chaos, all looked upon as perfection in retrospect of this living in hell or living in paradise. It is through these polarities that one gets to experience life, without them there would not be much to experience. Take the mind, clean its filing cabinet full of memories and beliefs out, at least for the moment and you will find yourself in the present.

It had been a wonderful time living with Rory and his family, a time to get to know each other a little better and become a part of their lives. There were memories of fishing salmon and cruising over the open Pacific on their boat. There were family gatherings sharing food and company in celebration as it should be. Enjoy each moment, they are but just a flash.

After a full day in Airports and planes, Traveler finally landing in Quito, Rishi anxiously awaiting. Once he cleared Customs and out the door into the Lobby, the search was on. It was like they had not seen each other in years, they both dropped to their knees in reverence for each other's presence, with teary eyes they just hugged, home again. Both were sharing stories and getting caught up with each other's experience of being apart, spending time alone. On the following morning they would journey back to the farm, resuming their life experience together.

Rishi had the property looking as if they had had gardeners working busily every day, the rose bushes with velvet red buds, yellow, white, and pink and well-groomed shrubs lining the driveway. At last, for the first time around their home they had a beautiful lush green lawn. A new walkway was in place leading from the garage to their house, everything looking perfect and ready to enjoy.

Their motorcycles were waiting to be taken out for a tour and enjoy the mountain air. It was back to the simplicity of life that exists in many parts of the Andes. This area boasts some of the best coffee grown in Ecuador, most nights in the village you can smell the beans being roasted and then freshly ground for their evening meal of humitas or tamales served with their favorite dark roast. The coffee is normally brought up from the farms by Burrow, hardly a day goes by that you don't see a loaded Burrow heading into el pueblo or returning home. At one time before the roads were in place, the trail down along the farm was a trade route between Peru and Southern Ecuador. With their wares packed these native Peruvians would load up the Burrows with their goods and journey for many days to reach this area in Catacocha where they would sell their merchandise. This traditional trade continues, with the exception that the burrows are used locally now, and trucks have taken over the long haul.

Traveler had many times remembered the words of the Yogis talking about the dark night of the soul and thought a few times that he had reached that moment when he would ask himself, "What the hell is this life all about?", but normally, after a few choice words, he would end up laughing at the mind, as it was willing to jump in any direction just don't lose me was its cry. The next year would bring quite a snack of dark days, hold fast...

Everyone has their own journey no way around it, each soul has its own truth to experience, only then can you call it your own and say that it is real. Rishi and Traveler prepared for their first ceremony on this farm and selected stones to be placed in a circle over the vortex in the living room. Once again, the four Cardinal points were determined, and specific stones placed to the North, South, East, and West and then the circle was completed by joining smaller stones together. Their ensuing ceremony was two-fold, one to celebrate the Solstice and the other was to open up the farm to be sold. The decision to sell the farm had been made when Traveler returned home, it is a feeling, you just have to go with it. From here on in Rishi and Traveler would try and allow life to present itself each day, easier said than done.

In January Rishi and Traveler began a methodology introduced by Alejandra from Argentina. Alejandra was in the final months of completing her unfoldment. Her work seemed to resonate with Traveler and Rishi so they both made a commitment to complete this unfolding of the Universal (higher Self), which would take over a year to complete. It is an in-depth exercise of bringing the Physical/Biological, Emotional, Mental, Soul and Distortional Planes into center or neutral. In a simple explanation it is bringing the past and the future experiences into present where they can be given to higher Self so that all may be put into order. The Word is order…

Their goal was the manifestation of higher Self directly into form so that this Intelligence is experiencing and guiding their moment to moment, I am presence.

There are ten quarantines to complete which are each forty days long. Each evening just before going to sleep, all of the day's events are given up to higher Self, once again so that that day can be put into order, one less thing for the mind to throw into dream time. No doubt about it, with the completion of each quarantine there was a shift in awareness. Rishi and Traveler were trying to remain centered or in the heart space each moment. Rishi was living it; Traveler was working at it. They were clearing memories and habits, some tougher than others to break and dissolve. In essence it was a continued effort to remove the interference so that their true nature could be experienced, definitely humor was returning.

Traveler decided to pitch a tent further down the mountain on the farm, so he could be alone and also to fast. Oh... that lonesome word, fast. He would stay there for three days, only herbal tea to drink if he felt like building a fire. The first night was not so bad, enjoy the stars and the sounds of wildlife stirring about, but the second and third day were like waiting for death or perhaps hoping for it. Traveler was committed to overcome this barrier that his mind had created, and he stuck it out. If nothing else, he had overcome the fear of being hungry or at least recognized it as another mind/body habit. Another Ceremony was done on the third night, this time over the vortex in the garage. Although Rishi was beginning to receive guidance each day from within, it was always good to be able to share experiences that they had during ceremony.

After a month or so they received guidance on a change of diet or the way that they were eating each day. They would only eat once a day and this meal would be eaten between 5:00 and 6:00 o'clock in the afternoon. Oh, Oh, Oh, there must be a better way, surely it was a miscommunication. Traveler cut a deal and he was allowed a little fruit and nuts at mid-day. It was the beginning of cutting out processed food, condiments etc. Catacocha has a huge street market of local growers on Sundays as well as their regular market throughout the week, so lots of fresh produce to choose from and as well fresh milled peanut butter ground daily.

To say that the next four months were tough would be an understatement for Traveler. It was one thing to be a little light on the groceries but couple that with the body detoxifying all those years of poor eating habits, especially in Ecuador, it was like dying a slow death. Traveler had to face the reality of not being able to do much outside work and spent more time in the house as his energy level was down. Hold Fast…

It was during these months that Rishi was receiving exercises to help them connect to the cosmic energy as well as to Mother Earth, and many exercises for their physical body. Their awareness was becoming more acute each week. There was no income so before long they were selling off whatever was not needed on the farm. After a couple of months, they were becoming more accustomed to the change in eating habits and now had a greater appreciation for their food. Their senses were becoming keener and beginning to realize what felt good to their bodies and what was depleting energy. Through their guides they were discovering what affects different food was having on them. Many days they thought how they could have been so asleep to all this information. It was far more in depth than any Health Clinic that Traveler had experienced during the past twenty years. Their bodies were changing dramatically, more tone and definitely leaner. Purification was taking on a whole new meaning.

Rishi and Traveler had enjoyed riding their motorcycles up and down the mountain roads, so much to discover. It was time for one of them to be sold, so whichever one went first, so be it. Things were getting pretty bare on the farm, but they knew that they were on the right path. Answers to their questions were coming much quicker, more and more they were connecting to their higher Self. One of Rishi's guides is an Apu named Upak who is from another dimension. An Apu on this plane is responsible for ceremonies for protection, connection to Mother Earth and Father Sun as well any other ceremony required within their communities. Upak had given them five places that they needed to visit as part of their spiritual journey. Traveler and Rishi were aware of this but were waiting for the farm to be sold before heading out. The farm had buyers in July and for some reason they kind of fell off the map. Upak appeared in Rishi's vision one August morning and asked why they had not started their journey; the time is now. Rishi shared Upak's words with Traveler and just kind of left it like that. It was about fifteen minutes into yoga that morning on the patio, overlooking the beautiful San Antonio valley when it became clear that they needed to make the trip. Traveler looked at Rishi and said, "Let's make a list of what to sell". Rishi was ecstatic and jumped for joy. Within four days they had cleaned out the house, the rest of the appliances, furniture whatever was not nailed to the wall was sold. Ecuadorians are rather good at bartering, but Traveler and Rishi had enough cash in hand to make the trip, which would cover two of the five destinations laid out by Upak.

It was trip day and at midnight they were on the bus heading for Peru. All was on plan until they arrived at the small border town of Macara, Rishi had not registered her new Cedula (National ID), and they would not permit her to enter into Peru. It was back onto a bus home, took the bags of the bus and within 15 minutes they were on another bus heading for Machala where she would be able to register her card. The office in Machala did the change within a couple of hours and by 10:30 that night they were heading South to Piura Peru.

Traveler and Rishi were in Piura early in the morning, so they were able to obtain good seats on a Cama-bus (almost like travelling 1st class) to Lima and at the same time reserved seats for Cuzco. They arrived in Cuzco rather rested as the buses were amazing, bathroom, movies and meals were served, definitely worth the extra cost of the tickets.

From Cuzco they managed to find a Van heading for Ollantaytambo, a beautiful small village originally designed and built by the Incas. They would spend a night there and try and find their guide in the morning. Upak said that their guide's name was Andres and that they would find him in this small tourist village which was situated not so far from Machu Pichu.

They asked around to the locals where the closest Indigenous Village was, and they were directed to an area at the edge of town where the Quechua arrived each day by Van.

A small number of them had shops in the village where they would sell their hand-made clothing and artisan work. It was just at the North side of the village where they encountered Andres. Their old Toyota Van pulled up to the side of the dirt street and ten or twelve Quechua men and woman jumped out ready for their day in the village. All of them were wearing their traditional dress, women with flaring pleated red skirts and embroidered blouses and the men with beige colored pants worn with a variety of different styled shirts. They all had the same form of beige round hat tilted off to one side of their head and tied on with a colored ribbon or some were designed with intricate bead work. These women had a bouquet of artificial flowers in the center of their hats, some well taken care of and some not.

Rishi and Traveler approached the driver and said that they were looking for a man named Andres, and he quickly answered, "I am Andres." or "Soy Andres." Traveler began to ask about his village and if they would be able to ride back with him when he was ready to return. They agreed upon a time and met back at the Van later that morning.

Their trip up the valley was like a step back in time, the mountains skirted with their stone terraces, which remained since the time of the Inca's. All of their small farms were being worked with teams of Oxen pulling their ploughs, no roar of the tractors here. These open fields were filled with color as the families picked stones or planted seed, springtime was upon them. It was a difficult climb for the old diesel Van, but finally it came to rest in their village, known as Huilloc. This village sits at around 4000 meters above sea level and yes it was fresh but thankfully it was sunny.

Although their tradition of sharing within their community and being in harmony with Mother Earth as well as their methods of working the land were well dated; this town had a fairly modern look and well maintained. It was similar to a small village in Ecuador, a variety of different colors on many homes, each having electricity and running water. Traveler and Rishi walked around the village for a while, Rishi wanted to make sure that they were in the right placed, find landmarks that she had seen in her vision.

They decided to stay with Andres and his family as their home was set up for guests or tourists. By late afternoon it was getting pretty cool, so they picked up their bags where they have left them earlier at one of the small stores and walked down to Andre's place.

Their guest room was simple, no form of heat but a good stack of blankets on standby. Traveler and Rishi joined Andres and his family in the kitchen for supper. Saturnina was cooking over the open fire inside the kitchen, it was a bit of an art as they had to leave the kitchen door open to get a good enough draft for the fire. Traveler and Rishi were feeling every hint of a breeze that came flowing down from the mountain. It did not seem to affect Andres or Saturnina in anyway, just laughing and sharing their day.

During supper they had a chance to ask about their Apu. Andres said that he had started out learning the ways of the Apu from his Father but opted for political duty and he had been elected as the Provincial Representative for the village. His father was not pleased with Andres, but the decision had been made. This area was home to three Apus that protected their valley, the village of Huilloc and Patacancha which was located higher up the mountain. They were highly respected by all the families in this valley and were always called upon for their ceremonies. These Apus are the spiritual guides to connect with Mother Earth, on behalf of the community. August was the month of giving back to Mother Earth and to the Apus for their work during the year. It was a perfect time for Traveler and Rishi to be there and to ask for a personal ceremony.

Andres said that the Apu living closest to them was named Domingo and he would talk to him later that evening to see if he could do a ceremony the following evening. As part of their tradition the Apu would walk the mountain looking for certain leaves and herbs to perform the ceremony. Domingo had asked Andres "What was the purpose of a ceremony for Traveler and Rishi", he was satisfied with their response and agreed to do the ceremony at Andres home.

Their first night in Huilloc was cool to say the least, Rishi and Traveler slept together in a single bed doing their best to get warm. They had both lost a lot of weight during the past year so there was no extra insulation on their bodies. Their stack of blankets over top of them was good for weight but a little too rigid to get tucked in properly around them. Going outside to the bathroom during the night was a major decision and not taken lightly but it was inevitable. When morning finally came, it was back to the kitchen for breakfast, hot tea was a welcome site. Saturnina served up corn pancakes, bread and jam which was well received, now they were ready for the day.

Rishi and Traveler did a little exploring of the valley and spent some time with different families in this community. Many of them shared their artistic work for Rishi and Traveler to see, some of it very impressive as it is all done by hand. There were quite a few small stone houses up the valley towards Patacancha sitting close to the river, all were abandoned. Andres said that they had been built after the Incas left but nobody in their village was interested in living in them. It did not seem to make sense to Traveler and Rishi as they both loved the idea of having a stone-built home.

Saturnina had returned from the field with their cattle and three children, the youngest strapped to her back. Andres was home from a day of travelling up and down the mountain with his Van. It was a great way for him to earn some money for the family, but it meant that his children and Saturnina had to manage the work at home and in the field.

Domingo arrived shortly after supper and set up his small altar in the room where Rishi and Traveler were staying. Andres joined in to translate for Domingo who only spoke Quechua. As he performed his ancestral ritual Rishi and Traveler were asked to select three leaves each leaf representing one of their spiritual guides. If the leaves were of good selection with no flaws this was a good sign that Mother Earth would favor the ceremony. Domingo takes his work seriously and wanted to make sure that Rishi and Traveler were serious about this ceremony as well. It was a ceremony meant to reconnect them to Mother Earth and be in harmony with her.

After the ceremony was completed Domingo quietly left carrying a cloth wrapped around their offering and headed up the mountain to a sacred place where it would be buried in the earth. Domingo prefers to walk alone as he said that you cannot look back and those on this sacred walk cannot have any fear as there are dark energies around who would take this offering for their own. It was done…

After a night short on sleep, the next day was spent with Andres and his family where they were working their Chakra (land used for planting corn, oats, etc.). Rishi and Traveler helped Saturnina carry lunch to the field which was wrapped up in a tablecloth. Their Chakra was in a small valley with a stream running through the center of the fields, many families worked their individual sections there. Inca buildings/ruins were still there, terraces on the mountainside as well as a small abandoned Church. Andres said that they had discovered skeletons in the caves on the mountain. They were a civilization who lived there before the Quechua. Their bodies were less than a meter high and it appeared as if they went into the caves to sit and permit the body to die because there was no sign of struggle or deformity. Traveler had seen quite a few people in Cuenca that were less than one meter in height. These people had difficulty stepping up onto the city bus and often required assistance, but other than their size their features were the same as what would be considered normal.

Saturnina served lunch, hot soap, and then laid the tablecloth open over the grass to display the buffet of potatoes, vegetables, and other traditional food. It was a moment of laughing and sharing, it seemed so perfect, what a way to experience life. Their oldest son managed to guide the plough after lunch and Saturnina helped to turn the Oxen around at the completion of each furrow. Their son was so happy to be old enough to run the plough. Up and down the hillside with her child on her back and Saturnina still had energy to laugh and play.

Rishi and Traveler definitely liked this simple way of living that Andres and his family enjoyed as part of this thriving community but from their perspective it was not an easy life. There were very few older community members working in the field, it is tough work. Each tribe or community had their benefits and burdens, Traveler and Rishi were in observation of these as they journeyed along. Their most important part of this journey was their committed connection to Mother Earth, Gaia/Mahii, anchored in this ceremony with Domingo. Although not totally clear to Rishi and Traveler, ceremony helps to bring the physical to the spiritual and vice versa so it is important to express through words on this plane and through intention so that the healing process can be carried out not only here but on all planes past, present and future, all present moments on each that are connected to Mother Earth. Intention is a key word as it holds power on what or where we hold our thoughts.

Early next morning Rishi and Traveler packed up their things and enjoyed one last breakfast with their host family before heading down the mountain road with Andres. The experience had been as their guide Upak had laid out for them, one only needs to follow their heart, and this was also part of their lesson to live more from their heart (connection). They reached Ollantaytambo and exchanged phone numbers with Andres in the event that their paths might cross again.

Within an hour or so they were on their way back to Cuzco where they could catch a bus to Bolivia. Urubamba is a beautiful City not too far from Ollantaytambo, it sits along el Rio Vilcanota in a huge valley much like an Oasis. Both Rishi and Traveler felt that it would be a wonderful place to live. These lush green valleys flowed gently down to the river and each valley with their own flow of fresh mountain water. They wound their way up the mountain road recapping the experience of the past few days, magical for sure.

Cuzco is quite a tourist center, so it was not long before they were on a bus travelling to Puno a city situated on the banks of Lake Titicaca. Traveler was never a big fan of buses, but these Cama buses gave a new meaning to the ride. If you can book the front seats on the second deck, it gives quite a vantage point to see the beautiful tapestry unfold in front of you. In August, Peru and Bolivia's Andes are still displaying their snow-white caps glistening in the sun, each curve of the mountain road winding your view closer and closer to their magnificence. Once they reached Puno Rishi and Traveler encountered an older Lady serving up a hot drink and homemade Arepas. This local hot drink called Champu was a first for Rishi and Traveler, it was brewed using corn, pineapple, and a few other spices. It was quite a treat and they made sure to find this Lady on the way back.

Their next leg of the journey took about ten minutes with their bags piled up on a three wheeled bicycle taxi, a 3.00 Soles ride to the parking area where a Van would take them to the border of Bolivia. It was another spectacular ride as the road to Desaguadero follows along the water's edge of Lake Titicaca. It is as beautiful as every description that Traveler and Rishi had read about before they set out on their adventure. Definitely another area where one could hang his hat for a while if life put the opportunity out there. Once they were in the border town, they loaded up their belongings on another Bicycle Taxi, the owner of this ride is a calm soul, so Rishi and Traveler took some time to enjoy his company and share a fresh fortified maca and fruit shake. This kind man waited for Rishi and Traveler to clear customs and also showed them where to get the best exchange on Soles to Bolivianos. It was a welcomed break for Traveler and Rishi after many hours of travel.

Being in Bolivia was a nice experience for Rishi and Traveler, the Bolivian people seem to be very accommodating, all looking to carve a daily existence out of life but only taking what they need. Often when tourists are drifting through, the thought pattern is take as much as you can from them, we will never see them again, but not so in these small communities of Bolivia.

Upak had directed them to Tiwanaku/Tiahuanaco where they would find their next contact. A taxi from the main highway drove them into this small Pueblo and the driver suggested a Hotel near the Central Park which turned out to be a good location for Rishi and Traveler. This Hotel was in the right price range and cost 70 Bolivianos per night or roughly $10.00USD for the both of them. It also had a small restaurant where the young owner and her father prepared the lunch specials and other meals. This restaurant was always full of many Quechua people and other locals who worked for the Municipal Offices as well as people working inside the Pyramid of the Sun. It turned out that the owner was associated with the Indigenous community and personally knew two of the local Apus. They planned to meet with one of them, later that night.

Clemente arrived at the Restaurant around 8 o'clock that night dressed in a couple of layers of ponchos as the nights drop below freezing. He is by far one of the humblest beings that they had ever met. He had a bit of Rishi's gift and was able to see things that many cannot. After they talked for a half hour or so he knew what ceremonies were needed to assist them on their spiritual path. They would wait until the following night to do their first ceremony as it was a better day of the week. Clemente explained that there are days of the week that are dark energy and not good for the soul to open up in ceremony. This initial ceremony time was set for the following evening.

Evening came and before long Clemente and his wife Ortencia were outside the Hotel ready to take them to the ceremony site. Rishi and Traveler had purchased all that was required for two separate ceremonies earlier that day with the guidance of Clemente. This store at one end of town had everything and more that had to do with sacred ceremonies. Into the darkness they began their long walk out of the village towards the South until they came upon a small footpath heading back towards the West. Clemente explained while they were leaving the village that there was a Guardian who would normally not permit access to this sacred spring where he wanted to do a purification ceremony for Rishi and Traveler. In the thirty-five years as an Apu he had only been to this spring twice before and had to pay money to the Guardian Anciana/Elder to permit a short meditation by the spring but no ceremony.

Others had tried to enter this sacred ground but within a short time they heard dogs barking and then this old Lady or Anciana was standing in front of them sending these people away. Clemente said that in reality those that know her say that she is almost blind and feels that she has powers to be able to move from one place to another. They all walked along the path in darkness, no flashlights allowed. They took the odd speed wobble as the path was difficult to stay on but eventually made it to the sacred spring. Clemente set up the ceremony and built a small fire. They use a sweet wine as part of the purification and it is thrown on the fire, not consumed. They were all sitting on the ground ready to connect to Mother Earth, when the energy started to flow up their tailbones it was like hot liquid rising up the spine, something Traveler and Rishi had never experienced, at least not to this extent. Clemente also had a cloth with leaves, similar to Domingo, that they needed to select for the offering, these would be placed in the fire. They all had very favorable visions which they shared before going to the spring's edge for purification, Clemente used this fast-flowing water to purify Traveler and then Rishi. You could definitely feel the presence of ancient civilizations and their Antepasados/Ancestors.

They gave their gratitude to Mother Earth for permitting their ceremony to be completed without interruption and started their walk back with lightness of body, mind, and spirit. Clemente felt that Traveler had been a Sacerdote in the time of the Pukinna Culture, which was before 500 AD. The Aimara Culture began around 500AD and continued until the Quechua/Inca era beginning in 1450AD. Ortencia gave Traveler and Rishi a short prayer to call upon Pacha Mama for purification of the heart. There were many things to share on their walk back to the village that night. Clemente not only came from a long lineage of Apus but also at this time he was working with the Archeology team on the grounds in and near the Temple of the Sun. His history was both scientific as well as teachings passed down from his Antepasados to confirm them.

One last ceremony, so the next morning Rishi and Traveler were out the door at 5:00 o'clock and into the darkness as they had to be in front of the Temple before Father Sun came up for the day. It was a cold walk in the pitch black with only the stars shining but they were excited about this ceremony. It was: The Birth of Father Sun (Tata Inti) and Mother Earth (Pachamama) within Rishi and Traveler. Sons of the Sun and Mother and the Cosmos giving Energy and Knowing to their consciousness.

Ceremonia: Nacimiento de Padre Sol y Pacha mama adentro Rishi y Traveler. Hijos del Sol y Madre y el Cosmos darle Energía y Conocimientos...

They met up with Clemente and Ortencia and walked up the hill not too far from the Gateway to the Temple of the Sun, in an area that had a few half walls or ruins. Clemente started a fire, this time he was able to build a much bigger one for the ceremony, no looking over their shoulders for the Anciana. Rishi and Traveler selected their offerings for Father Sun and Clemente spoke his ceremonial words. They all sat in meditation until Tata Inti began to rise over the mountain to the East, it was at that moment that they all stood up in reverence of his light and remained there with hands out facing the East for quite a while. Rishi and Traveler truly felt connected to Pacha Mama and Tata Inti and felt that they had retraced the lands of past lives, closing off the circle. Clemente definitely had a broader understanding of the cosmic connection with all forms of life here on Earth than his fellow Apu, Domingo, had demonstrated in Huilloc.

The Condor represents Tata Inti (Father Sun) the connection or energy of Ra. The Puma represents Mother Earth and symbolizes the Guardian of Earth. These two energies connected or unified bring the duality Masculine/Feminine together in a human being.

Cosmos/Spirit/Creator gives life to this form...

Clemente explained that what was left to view of the pyramid was only 18 meters above the ground level. Many stones of the pyramid were removed by the Spaniards to build the Walls in Tiwanaku as well as the Church in the center of the Village. One of the huge central Churches in La Paz was also built from these stones. Most of the pyramid is below the surface and is being studied by Archeologists along with Clemente at this time. Truths of these pyramids, their purpose and the ancient cultures that inhabited them, rarely comes to public knowledge, such a shame that those who want to control this world have to resort to these tactics, afraid that someone might wake up.

Their reign is coming to an end as each soul awakens to claim their power, their sovereign rights as a human being and co-creates a unified world without domination by another…

Traveler and Rishi walked back down the path with Clemente and Ortencia once again feeling quite light, connected, and full of energy. It was a wonderful space to be in. They said their good-byes to their Apu and his wife, gave their gratitude and each went on their way…

It was still quite early when they returned back to the Hotel, so they made a decision to take a Van to La Paz, the fare was within their budget. La Paz is a big city, feels a bit like Quito but fifteen years behind in growth or modernization. Traveler and Rishi were blessed, all of the downtown streets were closed to traffic that day, to permit an Indigenous demonstration. They were lobbying for higher wages and did this in a calm orderly fashion. It was wonderful to be able to walk the streets without the noise of traffic and the pollution that goes with it. They walked around for an hour or so and then took a ride up the mountain on the new Public Teleferico before heading back to Tiwanaku. They wanted to gather up their belongings in Tiwanaku and cross the border while there was still lots of daylight.

They reached Puno late that afternoon and reserved their seats for an overnight trip to Cuzco. It was time to liberate or give a new home to the sacred stones from the farm along with a few other significant stones and crystals. They flagged down a Moto-taxi and headed for the Lake, there Rishi and Traveler did a short ceremony before tossing the stones one by one into the lake, this was a moment they had been waiting for, for almost two years. Completing or closing this part of their life off felt pretty good. From there it was off to crash the diet and enjoy some pizza, Puno has quite a selection of Pizza Restaurants, so it was just a matter of choosing one.

Rishi and Traveler reached Cuzco the next morning and decided to spend a day there and then board the bus back to Lima the next morning. They wanted to take in the scenic drive during daylight and were able to book the front seats on the 2nd level once again.

They took a taxi to the Terminal and their day started out pretty well but by nightfall, and still on the bus, Traveler was sicker than a small dog, and searching for plastic bags to empty out the body. A bus winding down the mountain road is not the ideal place for a slow death but one has to hang on. He was afraid to close his eyes for fear that the other unsuspecting eye… might open and fill his trunks. That is living in fear.

Traveler and Rishi made it to Lima in one piece, happy to be outside once again. Cuzco to Ecuador is a long haul, no doubt about it, but they kept at it. They crossed the border into Ecuador about Noon the next day and still had about $30.00 in their pocket, so it was a good trip. Neither Rishi nor Traveler have a credit card for back up so trust in Creator is a must.

It was great for Traveler and Rishi to be back on the farm, nothing really changes, peace and quiet hold their place. Now the reality of no furniture and no appliances had settled in. Traveler always liked making a fire, so that became the daily chore, gives a whole new understanding of keeping the home fires burning. They figured if Saturnina could do it so could they. Before long Traveler hammered out some tin to make an oven so that they could bake bread. They made their own culture, not wanting to use yeast. This artisan bread was exceptional to say the least. There was also homemade chocolate cooked with Manteca de cacao (butter of the Cocoa) and a little raw sugar.

They quickly adapted to living without any source of power or cooking appliances. In Ecuador Traveler and Rishi did not look out of place, many neighbors lived this way but if they tried that in Canada they would quickly be labeled as hippies, better get a job. Some days Traveler and/or his mind would have liked to bail out and head to Canada again to step back into the world, but both he and Rishi knew that they needed to continue a little deeper into their process.

Within a month they sold the rest of the garden equipment and headed to Quito where they rented a small space to live for a month (no furniture). They wanted to experience the big city to see if their understanding was real or just something that they experienced on the quiet of their farm. They also wanted to spend some time with Victor who was now working in Quito. They slept on cushions on the floor for that month and cooked all meals with a rice cooker, Rishi can put magic into a simple meal.

There were lessons to be learned. First out the gate was all the attractions that were available for the mind. There were shops full of new clothes, shoes, hats and every imaginable luxury to enjoy. Gringo Town, which is located in Quito's city center, offers a wide variety of Restaurants for dining out, what delicacies… It was a treat to let the mind out, but it was soon in line once again, in harmony and balance, not affecting their experience one way or the other, just remaining in center, in neutrality, well almost.

Quito has a number of homeless people, Gypsies, street musicians etc. It was a time to reflect on their lives and how they approached each day. Traveler failed a couple of tests, one day with the last twenty dollars in their pockets an older gentleman dressed in a suit come to their side in tears. He needed money to be able to buy his wife's medicine. He asked for twenty dollars, how could he have known that that was all that Traveler and Rishi had in their possession. Yes, the mind took a little kick at the cat in disbelief of the story, but that was not the point. Quickly return to neutrality, Traveler looked at Rishi and said, "We could do ten." The man was crying in gratitude, Traveler said to Rishi, "I know, we should have given him the twenty." she just smiled. Rishi has no fear of giving her last bit of plata as they call it in Ecuador. Traveler had a way to go to reach that level of understanding.

Their next opportunity to let go was a few days later in the park close to their apartment, (Elejido Parque). They had received another small payment on the generator from a man at home who bought it and had that same amount in the pocket again, twenty dollars. This time it was one of the older Gypsy gals who played the part. She asked Rishi for twenty dollars to do a special little ceremony for abundance of life, for her and Traveler. Traveler could only see the insanity of this moment, but Rishi had seen the real reason why, she is the Seer. There was a debt owed to this woman from another lifetime. This opportunity had now presented itself to pay the debt. Traveler handed over the twenty dollars and felt like ploughing part of the park with his feet but refrained, (kind of like a temper tantrum). As his father so often said, "Nothing good to say better to say nothing." Traveler knew that he could not stay in silence for long, Rishi and he were beyond that. After a few minutes Rishi shared what had passed and all was good, back to living lean, real lean. Thank God for rice at forty-nine cents a pound.

Traveler and Rishi had not eaten much food outside of their home for a long time, so their bodies were becoming more detoxified as the months went on. As one experiences life with a little more awareness the lessons turn into knowing and understanding as the evolution of the soul continues.

Their focus was to stay in their heart or center, it is in that space where questions can arise and answers can be received, not from the mind but from your eternal wisdom. The sensitivity to certain foods was the next lesson. It soon became clear that all condiments were like a drug additive which changed the vibration of the body. It would require a lot of explanation to go over the amount of poison that actually is put into food preservatives, processed wheat, wheat, processed salt, sugar, and the list goes on. Just the few aforementioned are contained in most food that is sitting on the grocery shelves. As Ramana said, "It is as it is".

The human race has free will, they have a choice whether to experience life in a lower vibration or frequency and permit all the programming, radiation, poisoning etc. that is being offered as real food. If it is not taken from a tree, plant or out of the earths soil, then it is going further and further away from being good for you. It maybe is not that simple but that is each person's discovery. Become aware of what big business is doing to the human race as a whole here on Mother Earth, profit is the word. It is comfortable, just like sleeping in a warm soft bed, nobody wants to get out of it and that is alright, but if you are sufficiently tired of your experience then awaken from your sleep. It will be tough, there are many seemingly conveniences in this world, but we do not have to be fooled by all of them, your power is much greater than that, always was and always will be…

Quito had given Traveler and Rishi what they needed to expand their awareness; life is a game, but it changes when one is playing a little more consciously. They had discovered a few good sources in Quito, of organic grains, nuts and produce and were able to implement new recipes into their diet which were very agreeable to their bodies. It takes an effort to change the daily habits one only needs to be consistent and open to make these changes. It was time to return to the farm and put their new knowledge into practice and continue to listen to their guidance from within.

Back to the farm and back to the basics of cooking with fire. Traveler liked to build big fires and use the hot coals as required, but they had depleted the wood piles into the danger zone. The rainy season was starting so it was necessary to move the fire pit under the garage roof and also bring in a supply of wood that was stacked up in another part of the farm, ready… Traveler and Rishi remembered Saturnina cooking over a small fire, so Traveler adapted and made the change. It was quite a bit quicker and definitely there was less consumption of wood. There is a bit of freedom or independence when one knows that they can live well and simply without electricity and all the modern conveniences. In reality Rishi and Traveler lacked for nothing.

Over the next few months there were many days without a dime in the ole cookie jar, but they never missed a meal. If one allows Creator to look after your well-being, He never falters. Confidence in Him is not so easy to come by, He wants that confidence in Him to be unshakeable, there needs to be a letting go (of being in control). Just relax in knowing, that He is there, never left, only the interference of the mind got in the way. Each soul has his own truth to discover, his own way of returning back to Source, that is the adventure.

Not long after they had arrived home Traveler and Rishi had the same vision, Traveler brought it up one morning a couple of days later and Rishi confirmed that she had had the same vision. They saw themselves standing on the driveway at the bottom of the hill about twenty meters away from the house. They were standing in front of a medicine wheel made from stones and around the medicine wheel was another circle of stones. Mother Earth appeared later that day inside their home in the form of a huge black Puma sitting on her haunches, her head almost touching the beams at four meters. Rishi sat down in that space to connect with Mahii.

Rishi had lit a candle and an incense, Mahii asked what that smell was, Rishi replied that it was an incense, Mahii shook her snout in disapproval. Mahii said that Cedar, Palo Santo, and Copal are proper incense, which can be found in Ecuador. Mother Earth explained to Rishi that the medicine wheel was to open up a vortex that would bring balance and harmony to the climate in and around the area, West towards Loja, and South towards Peru.

This ceremony would be performed the next day in the exact spot they had seen in their vision. Rishi and Traveler would have to stay on the farm for three days afterwards. A soft rain would begin on the third day and then in intervals that she indicated would happen over the following couple of months. It would take quite a while to bring balance back to the area as there are many things involved at other levels of understanding which Traveler and Rishi were not yet aware of.

Rishi and Traveler selected stones and built the medicine wheel which is about three meters in diameter and then the outside circle of stones was placed within a five-meter diameter. This outer circle of stones is protection given by Creator. Their ceremony was set to begin at 4:00 o'clock in the afternoon, at which time they would have a large fire burning not too far from the medicine wheel.

As the Ceremony unfolded so did the story behind the reason that Rishi and Traveler were living on this farm. Mahii appeared in the form of Kundalini a large white Serpent and Father Sun was present in the form of cosmic energy; they are our brothers and sisters as is all life within first Source.

It was shown that Traveler was one of the seven brothers who held dominion over the Paltas tribe which extended far into Peru and around the Western part of the province of Loja, reaching out in all directions. With the arrival of the Incas into the Paltas region, it was to be the end of the brother's reign over their land. Traveler was the spiritual leader of the Paltas Nation in this period of time. A pact was eventually reached with the

Incas where they would allow the seven brothers to maintain their reign but under the direction of the Incas.

Soon the Incas were requesting that the seven brothers kill off some of their fellow tribesmen who were posing a threat. This act of killing was not part of the original agreement. After a short while the seven brothers rebelled but to no avail, they were over-powered and brought up to Shiriculapo to be burned at the stake. Peña de Shiriculapo is a rock formation that stands close to 300 meters in height and acts as a cliff. Before their death, the seven brothers under the guidance of Traveler put a curse on their own land so that it would not produce for the Incas. During the time of the Paltas this land produced 100% of the time during the year so it was an area of abundance. The slaughter of Paltas men and children continued until there was hardly a trace of them in this region.

At this point of the ceremony performed for Mother Earth, there were six Paltas brothers who appeared and stood on the outside of the medicine wheel. They were there to receive guidance from Traveler whose energy had remained partly in the Astral Plane since their death. It was time to remove the curse and return home in peace, bringing harmony and balance to this area once again. His brothers were waiting for Traveler to give them instructions on how to enter the vortex. Traveler went into a bit of a conscious trance and began to chant and sing the ancient song along with a mudra formed with his hands.

Rishi was able to see and know all that was happening, she asked Traveler on another plane why he was using this mudra as she understood it to hold dark powers. Traveler/Paltas replied that the mudra can be used for either light or darkness. Rishi said that the six brothers were waiting for their final step. At that moment Travelers arms went out to each side and felt the connection of his brothers. In an instant Traveler felt like his body was shrinking almost ten times smaller until the moment that the seven were returned to the vortex.

This ceremony had now closed a chapter of the Paltas tribe and their seven leaders, bringing the beginning of balance and harmony to the climate. A purification needed to correct an imbalance created over five hundred years prior. Their huge fire was part of this purification for the Earth and for the healing of these seven Paltas brothers. It was also a moment of purification for Rishi and Traveler as they continue to purify their connection with Great Spirit (Creator) which has been hindered by their mind/ego, not only in this life experience but in past lifetimes. Each step since the Amazon to Peru, Bolivia and here in Paltas are all connected.

Traveler and Rishi had visited Shiriculapo, a high bluff on the West side of Catacocha, and felt its dark energy trying to pull them closer to the edge. It was this Cliff where the Paltas were thrown to their death by the Incas. Many couples and other people had fallen to their death while standing on Shiriculapo, the local folk thought that it was some kind of love energy attracting couples, not to be… At the bottom of the cliff is a portal, inside this portal is like a city of astral beings searching to feed on the light, as they had lost their way home to Source.

Not too long after this Ceremony there was a huge fire on Shiriculapo which bellowed black smoke high into the sky until it had burned the face of Shiriculapo clean. This was a purification of these dark energies as well. During the time that the three vortexes were opened on the farm, there were many astral beings that came to find these portals and return home. There are many imbalances here on Mother Earth that need to be returned to peace, harmony and balance. As each soul takes responsibility for their own purification process this assists greatly in healing Mother Earth and humanity. She will guide you in one form or another if you ask and are serious enough to do what it takes. Do not ask half heartily, as the Sages have said more or less "Better not to start the spiritual path but if you do, better complete the work."

THE FINAL CEREMONY

Experiencing life on the farm was a gift in every aspect. Looking out from their home were the Andes, these mountains appeared like a carpet of lush green trees protecting the native flora and small communities throughout the valley below. It is wonderful to breathe in this oxygen filled air free from pollution of any kind. It was an Ashram for Traveler and Rishi, and they know in their hearts what a blessing it was to live this experience and continue learning how to connect to Mother Earth. Traveler and Rishi were able to practice their salutations to Father Sun in the morning and in the evening just before setting behind the mountains. Our sun's rays are necessary to assist in the transformation of our DNA strands during this shift of consciousness on our planet. It is also a time of healing during the first rays of each new day flooding over the earth and the last rays before the Sun sets.

Over the next few months Rishi and Traveler would be open to a deeper understanding of food and its effects on the health of body/mind/spirit. They were living in absolute trust that life would unfold each moment of each day without any conscious effort from the mind, just being open to what Life presented to them. Remaining in their hearts, yes… Traveler still had a way to go but the percentage of time being centered was increasing each day.

When one is connected and experiencing existence more in observation from one's higher self, the outside world has little effect on the soul. There is still chaos going on in the world and in the mind space of many, but it has little or no power over the daily experience. Their minds were beginning to quiet, not being pulled out and reacting to every movement or situation. One does not normally see the difference from the outside but only from the individual perception of the soul within. This conscious looking out, changes and continues to change.

Each day Traveler and Rishi were asking Mother Earth for guidance so they could assist in some way in the healing of our planet and for guidance on how to heal themselves. Their variety of daily diet was getting narrowed down. Their shopping list was vegetables, fruit (mostly bananas and oranges, locally grown of course), plantain (five dollars buys enough for the week) and three pounds of fresh ground peanut butter at a dollar fifty per lb. Molloco is cooked plantain (more ripe than green) and peanut butter mixed together. Molloco is a staple food for locals and also for Traveler and Rishi for many months.

Segundo was a neighbor of Traveler and Rishi's, kind of their hero. He and his wife live down in the Valley where their farms adjoined. There was only a foot path leading down to Segundo's farm which was fairly steep in places with huge boulders along the trail, many would bail out halfway thinking that they could not make it back up to the main road. Segundo walks that trail each day with his burrows like he was a young man twenty five years old, he was eighty-eight at that time. He was as strong as a horse and was always smiling or laughing. His meals consisted of whatever grains he grew on the farm as well as fruits, vegetables, organic eggs, and a bit of rice, when he had some money. Segundo accepted his decision to live on a small farm that was difficult to reach, this simple life that it offered, but never complained. Traveler and Rishi looked at the health of Segundo, his stamina and outlook on life, it was admirable to say the least.

Segundo had a very touching way of saying goodbye to people he loved. He would raise his hands above his shoulders to indicate his connection to a higher power or God and then bring his hands down to cross over his heart and finally outwards to the people in front of him. Always with a tear of emotion, raw love from Source.

There are many further into the mountain area that live similar to Segundo, and many have had grandparents who lived to well over one hundred or a hundred and twenty years of age. Up the mountain road to where people were living in the village it was a different story, lots of restaurants cooking roasted chicken (six weeks from the chick to the table), res or beef and a favorite for the locals was chancho or pork. It is a whole other story on the dangers of eating the aforementioned buffet of carne (meat), thanks to injected hormones, medicated/balanced feed which is loaded with animal protein as opposed to plant protein. Unfortunately, when farmers look to become more profitable, they are educated by the feed companies on which products give the best results for growth, less days to market. It is in the best interest of the farmer to make a good living but many of them are not educated on the lethal cocktail that they are putting into the food chain. We all have a choice whether to support this practice or find a farm that understands the importance of remaining true to nature.

Rishi and Traveler continued on their path trying to fine tune their diet so that their purification process could continue. They were getting close to the last couple of months of their methodology and decided to cut the last bit of processed food out, and that meant no more homemade bread, at least until they would be able to grind their own flour. Traveler had stopped drinking coffee almost a year prior, big decision and he could argue in favor of staring the day with this tasty ritual, but it was just a decision. As much as possible they were trying to make their bodies available for changes in vibration. Mother Earth had been receiving cosmic energy for quite a while assisting Her and all life in this planetary change. There were many evenings when Traveler and Rishi could see the waves of energy going into the earth, about every five minutes usually starting just after dark and continuing until eight o´clock at night. The scientific world called it a plasma around the earth, it is cosmic energy here to assist with the graduation or ascension process of our planet.

As they became more in tune with their energies and ongoing changes, they were also becoming more aware of the quality of food and more conscious of their selections. Almost each week they had an opportunity to spend a day on other farms usually within an hour or so of their home. Each small farm had their fruit trees, herbs and banana plantations etc. When an orange, without chemical spraying, is picked from the tree there is life energy in that fruit, it could be felt from the first bite and right on into the stomach. Those experiences on each homestead seemed like an ideal way to live, interestingly enough many of these folks were looking to move into town for an easier life. On a small-scale hobby farm, it is hard work and for sure the body tires, where is the balance…

Each new day brought a more focused intention on eating with purification in mind and as well maintaining in their heart space. Yes, Rishi was still there… It was in that space that she received all of her guidance. Traveler was in quiet time one morning when he heard the ole voice again. Perhaps his uncertainty about the heart or center was floating around the cosmos, maybe…. The voice said quite simply, "I am the first breath, and I am the last". In that instant Traveler could feel the coolness of breath in his chest area, breathing in and breathing out. Creator might have been getting worn out trying to make it simple for Traveler, here was a sure way to stay centered, surely he would catch on.

It would not take a rocket scientist to figure it out, without breath there is no life. A newborn takes in the first breath and voila, life experience in the human body begins outside the womb, on the other hand when the body exhales its last breath, voila, it is the end of life for that human body. Traveler does not remember the name of the spiritual teacher, but his only teachings were these words: "Love is God, God is Breath within." Why all the lifetimes of spiritualty, the eons of meditation and studying to reach a moment when one of the most profound methods that really has significance, is to remain in your heart or center and be conscious of your breath.

Where is it…? If you placed a small triangle at the base at your sternum and the apex about 3 inches high pointing up towards your chin, that would about do it. Inside the hollow of your chest is where you exist, the soul connected to the back of your physical heart giving it the spark of life and the space around the soul is that connection to all that exists, the pathways the doorway, the Way back home to that Intelligence that gives life, that is Life. It is the connection between the physical world outside and the worlds, Universes and Galaxies within. Here is where the Son/Sun of the Sun resides, the Divine essence that all souls are, that brilliance of Light that has no bounds. It is in this space where all else ceases to exist, the game outside pales in comparison, but yet we long for the adventure.

Is it necessary to drag this looking for Self out for a lifetime…? Are many of the so-called spiritual teachers or Masters stuck in the rut of tradition, maybe… One thing is for sure if you can feel your center and can begin to spend as many present moments there as possible, all else that is required will come to you… There will be effort needed to purify the body/mind through clearing of the memories, beliefs and habits and through elimination of many foods, the latter normally happens of its own accord. Once again, the breath, be conscious of it. Wingmakers have a number of techniques to help remain in or open the connection to Source. Breathe in and make a conscious pause of your breath, you are there, in union.

Rishi was now a few months into her first seven months of spiritual training on another level or dimension. Their next spiritual guide is from Guatemala, another Apu. In reality the three Apus, Peru, Bolivia and Guatemala are an extension of Upak, experiencing life on the physical plane of Mother Earth.

Her training was received in a heart space mostly at night but sometimes during the day. No questions could be asked by Traveler so that no disruption would come to her mind. One question can cause a sequence of answers with the mind searching for them. Silence has many benefits.

During her first few days of being in form in this Guatemalan Indigenous village she was able to witness a ceremony, far beyond anything that she or Traveler had experienced in this lifetime. This tribe is quite consciously advanced and add a whole new meaning to devotion. Their ceremony was performed to assist Mother Earth in her ascension to the fourth dimension, by bringing in energy from other Star Planets. Their ceremony was being performed on other Planets at the same time which in turn were sending their intention of Light to Mahii/Earth. This ceremony began at four o'clock in the morning, no one in the village eats for twenty-four hours until the end of the ceremony the following day. Only children under the age of two years old, who as of yet do not have an understanding on the reason for fasting, can eat. Each of the tribal members have a natural gift that they were born with, some play musical instruments, some sing chants, some sing harmonic sounds, and some beat a drum to the rhythm of Earth's heartbeat.

This ceremony was done in precision and in synchronization with the other Star Planets. Around each huge fire walked the singer of the Mantras, seven turns one way and then seven turns the other way until one hundred and eight turns were completed. Each mantra being sung in harmony with the beat of the drum(s), the singing of sacred sounds which represent seven colors and the seven chakras. They continued without stopping for twenty-four hours and the wood fires were maintained to keep the connection open to the other Star Planets.

At four o'clock the next morning the Ceremony stopped at which time small wood fires were burning in front of each door of their homes whether it be Teepee or Adobe. They all sat on the ground to enjoy food that had been prepared and also to connect to the new energy that was now present on Mother Earth. Few people on our planet would be aware of this ceremony and its significance, our world news does not seem to focus on sacred events.

Within a few days Traveler and Rishi made plans for a similar ceremony in gratitude for their experience here on Mother Earth and also for a deeper purification of their spiritual process. Their guides suggested that Rishi and Traveler select at least three of their most favorite items to place in the fire to symbolize the letting go of attachments, they laughed as they did not have much left to get rid of. All of the clothes that they had left would fit in one suitcase. Interestingly enough they did have three things each that they liked a lot, for Traveler it was a favorite pair of shoes, a one-of-a-kind hand braided belt (so comfortable) and a good quality shirt that he had bought in Canada. Let go…

Their ceremonial fire was lit at 3:45 in the morning, the large stack of wood had been prepared the day before and covered in the event that it might rain. It was a good high blaze reaching 3 meters into the darkness, definitely a proper purification fire. At

4:00AM Traveler started his walk around the outside circle of stones that were placed around the medicine wheel while keeping beat on the drum. Following the example of their brothers and sisters in Guatemala he continued walking seven rounds one way and seven rounds the other. It was not long before the beat of the drum was changing and taking on a rhythm of its own. Rishi was sitting by the fire chanting in gratitude for this moment. Shortly after, at 4:30 Rishi sensed and saw other beings arriving to this ceremony, she began to take photos of their brothers and sisters in their light form (orbs).

Just before sunrise, at 5:30 Traveler and Rishi, separately, each placed their three favorite items into the fire and asked for purification or removal of all other things that were hindering their spiritual process. After that moment they went to sit in meditation within the circle of stones, Rishi facing to the South and Traveler facing to the North. From this point on other great beings took their place in this ceremony, Upak said that this moment was a gift from Great Spirit. Upak sat to the right of Traveler, Manu (Protector) sat facing East, next was Babajii, Rishi facing South, Shela (Guide), Amoon (In elephant form) facing West and in between her and Traveler was seated the Apu from Guatemala. Standing on the outside of the circle at the four directions were Arch Angel Michael, Uriel, Gabriel, and Rafael. Arch Angel Metatron was holding space over the medicine wheel vortex. Mahii and Tata Inti were there in energetic form.

In honor of their presence during this special moment in time, Traveler and Rishi bow down in reverence to their brothers and sisters who so graciously joined in on what would be the final ceremony on the farm, at least for Traveler and Rishi to perform.

How does one put it all together? Is there a short cut? Why bother with any of this? Maybe there is a short cut, but the underlying yearning needs to be towards awakening to the truth, your truth. It is from there (knowing who you are) that one can begin the adventure towards home. There are many who are so comfortable in this 3D dimension that they are not ready to leave it behind and that is okay… There are many who are sick and tired of the daily routine but never think that there might be something else to life, a more peaceful experience.

If we believe everything that we see each moment outside of ourselves, then we truly are living in an illusion. Yes, there is no doubt that it feels and appears real, but we need to know our own truth so we can decipher what is truly going on around us. These choices are ours to make each moment in this human experience here, and we do get pulled in by the illusion from time to time, not to be concerned because it is part of the adventure.

Traveler had a yearning since a fairly young age to search for some hint of truth in his life. He knew that hard physical work and drinking beer were not the key to a long enjoyable, healthy life experience. Internet was just taking off in the mid-nineties and new age books were hitting the shelves in the bookstores, it was a start. There is certainly a buffet of information available to anyone on their search, asking for guidance from within, will always bring you towards your truth much quicker than just searching aimlessly.

There are many consciously aware souls here on earth that are connected to other dimensions and able to bring these valuable teachings to those who are ready and open to receive. It is easier now to get to this point of awakening, the days of being a Yogi in the cave is not really required. Many headed for the cave to be in silence but also it became difficult to communicate with the outside world as their perception and understanding had changed.

Be aware while you are searching in that ocean of information streaming from the Internet, if it does not resonate with your soul, leave it. If there is anything in this story that does not feel right, do not try and believe it, just leave it… Each soul at some point in their lifetime is searching for their own truth and in reality, it is necessary to experience it before you can call it your truth. If there is one thing that has maintained its value down through the ages, it is meditation or being in silence with yourself, (Traveler's perception) that firm connection to Mahii/Mother Earth, (as these bodies or vehicles belong to this planet) and through our sun Tata Inti, which is fondly known by the Apus as our cosmic connection. To be quiet with yourself and disconnected from your thoughts, is to be connected to Source.

When you are in alignment with Source, you are at peace and in calm, and when you are not your thoughts pull you away, off into disharmony. As is indicated by the Wingmakers, living your experience in alignment with the wisdom path, sovereign integral. Yes, your higher Self can manifest directly through you if and when you are consciously available to receive Its guidance.

It seems like extremes are a prerequisite to this adventure we volunteer for here on earth. Perhaps it a way of broadening the experience so that one has completely satisfied the desires of the senses, nothing left untouched. It is through discovering all of the extremities that one can get a sense of where balance lies and how to return to it. Many of these extremes can feel painful and others enjoyable but if one can remain with peace of mind through those experiences then we can be more balanced in our approach to life.

Be with yourself/Self, do not have any fear of the unknown, it can be uncomfortable for the mind, but it is the ego/mind that each person needs to quiet or put to rest. Your goal is to become consciously aware of who and what you truly are. Our experience here on earth can be an adventure that builds character for our soul, but for many it can feel like a life full of despair. Do not be discouraged by the mind's flow of thoughts, be assured that you can quiet them by being conscious of your breathing. As mentioned by Thoth the Atlantean, the Word is Chaos that can be brought into Order. This is the work of the soul, taking the distortion out of the experience through purification of body/mind and the memories and beliefs held in your present moment or experience.

Emotional abuse does not leave any physical marks, but it leaves memories that one might unknowingly be very protective of, keeping them buried deep. There is no need to feel shame or guilt, blaming yourself or another as this will only keep you stuck in a painful experience. You may need help to let these memories go, ask for guidance from within and the right person will be directed to you, do not give up. Love always comes into the equation, in truth It is always present, but the confusion arises when we try to categorize this essence/feeling in relationship to those around us.

We first need to love ourselves, without self-love there is little chance of genuinely loving another, and less likely to love someone who may have caused us harm or unconsciously inflicted this pain on you. In reality many of the memories are from other lifetimes, reoccurring in this lifetime and waiting to be cleared. Once again, it normally takes guidance, at least in the beginning of your process, to recognize what memories are coming to the surface, ready to be released.

Massage therapy, Reflexology, Reiki, Acupuncture and Acupressure can all be a benefit in bringing health to the body/mind and open up the meridians so that the physical, mental and spiritual can begin working in harmony and balance. Once you have learned how to bring these memories up and clear them, then you can do most of the work yourself, in reality you are doing all the work. Memories come up as pain or as a feeling or energy that might surface when someone (maybe your spouse or partner), has trigged it by some comment. Your partner can be the gift, the opportunity to dig deep and find out where the agitation is coming from. That is the moment to get in tune with this feeling and find out where it is arising from. Eventually you become more aware of a feeling or energy arising and recognize that it is an opportunity to release it rather than be overwhelmed by it.

Be aware of your food intake and become knowledgeable on what is agreeable with your body, do not assume that our food sources are equally as nutritious as they were back in the fifties before GMO, herbicides, pesticides, and grains such as wheat that have been modified. As our consumers become programmed during this changeover to plant-based foods, awareness becomes even more important. Just because it tastes delicious does not mean that it is healthy for your body. Each human body is different, sure they can adapt but some seem to function well on vegan foods and others need meat or fish protein to keep the right amount of muscle mass and energy.

Traveler asked his neighbor one day about his farming practice which included growing GMO soybeans with the use of a chemical called Round-up that kills all plant life above the surface of the earth. His neighbor said that there was no need to worry, the soybeans were only for animal use, which meant that the beans would be fed to his cows for milk production and of course for his beef cattle. Neighbor was still a little bit asleep; he did not follow the food chain any further than the milking parlor. It does actually get much worse than this when you consider that animal protein is fed to animals/chickens in order to provide protein in their feed rations.

Organic is good but not all that is labelled organic is organic. The more you know about the source of your food the better, follow it back to the farm if you can, better yet, buy from the farmgate. The easiest method for eliminating something from your diet is: if you cannot understand the names of the ingredients on the label then there is an exceptionally good chance that it is not good for the body...

Do not avoid your pain by trying to cover it up with medication or by putting it off until another day. Recognize this energy that is with you, it is coming up to the surface for a reason. Take the time to deal with it by finding the source or sources of this memory, live it once again in your mind space, give it a feeling of love, let it go and begin the healing… If you put it off it will come back with much more force the next time. Rishi was dedicated and still is, at being in the moment to be with her pain, she has a clear understanding that it is her right and responsibility to take the time to release it. It is also your right…

Call it as you wish, being present, being in your center, being in your heart space, whatever feels right to you, that is where one needs to begin to become conscious of. Life as a human being is to experience the world in all of its simplicities and complexities, if we remain connected to the past it is difficult to raise your experience to another level of consciousness. Your mind can be a great tool to assist in your ascension journey or expansion of consciousness, so take control of it. Slowly or quickly, one pulls the attention away from the outside world and becomes aware of their being, their presence, the I am Presence of the present here and now… Being aware of the breath in this heart space as its cool freshness flows in and out, is one of the ways that Traveler uses to stay connected to Source. Find your Way…

All of life flows out from your heart and leads back to it. Creation and our part in co-creating caused confusion in Traveler's experience many times. He knew that we all have the power to co-create but at this level of understanding there seemed to remain a question as to whether one remains in neutrality in center or steps out to some future plan or creation. It took a while, almost twenty years, but clarity seemed to present itself not so long ago. Remaining in your heart or center is definitely the first step, being in that flow of wisdom will place all other necessities aside. There is a great responsibility in the power of creating as all thoughts (negative or positive) have possibility, so as long as there are negative thoughts flowing in our minds, it is best to try and remain in neutrality. There is a grand Idea for Life, which includes all of creation, so be in alignment with that Idea and live your life's experience by the will of your Source. Thy Will Be Done.

Be open to receive assistance from your guides who are waiting for your permission. One could repeat the following before going to bed:

"Dear Creator, I open myself to receive your light and all assistance possible for my healing and transmutation. I open up my heart, my soul, this body and mind for purification. May all assistance be given for the higher and greater purpose of All."

Laugh and laugh some more, do not take yourself to seriously, give as much attention to your spiritual nature as possible but keep the feeling light, not like it is a work activity. In the Airport in Vancouver Traveler was caught with his pants down so to speak. Maybe it was the news that he received that day that his father had passed away that caused a little confusion in his mind or perhaps the yellow caution sign that said the floors are wet at the entrance of the bathrooms. Whatever caused this lapse of attention it gave way to entering the Woman's Washroom. He should have caught on when he did not see any Urinals lining the wall, but he dismissed that final opportunity to clue in and proceeded to enter the second last stall in a row of at least fifteen.

There at last not a soul in sight, privacy with his pants down resting on the floor. From that lowered point of view, he could see a pair of Lady's shoes to his left in the next stall over. There was an instant bead of perspiration that caused quite a flush over the body, oh no… Decision time, too late, there was an influx of women and judging from the chatter and slamming of the stall doors, at least five or six in this group. Thoughts of pervert were skating through his mind, 911 was still fresh on the news and Airport security was a little more alert. Almost a nervous laughter arose within him as he thought if I ever get out of here, I will have to share this story with Jimmy. Traveler waited until all was quiet and walked out as quickly and as calmly as possible, only one woman was busy washing her hands at the sink, she caught the shadow behind her, but no screaming. Out in the lobby it seemed like everybody was waiting for Traveler's exit, but for sure a group of teenagers had seen him going into the wrong washroom and were killing themselves laughing in anticipation of what would happen. Laughter is good…

"See Yourself Happy" "Be Happy"

Traveler made the error (supposedly there are no errors) of being too caught up in this ole holy spiritual life. The ego is slippery, it will try and claim anything as it's own. It is designed as a protective mechanism but not designed to take control of your life. Traveler's life experience up until he was thirty-five or so was laughter, yes lots of pain, but the laughter was always there to heal. After thirty-five years, perhaps the pain had started to knock the wind out him and fewer moments for laughter remained. Don't let that happen, give it all that you can if that's what you feel in your heart but keep it light and enjoy each moment of the journey, laugh at yourself for being serious, laugh at life for being able to take you to the ground every once and a while. Get up in knowing that this Great Spirit or Source has designed this game of life here on Earth and beyond, trust that IT is only a breath away…

I AM ∞ WE ARE This Wonderous Life

NOTES

NOTES

NOTES